SANDPLAY

Kalff, Dora M.
    [Sandspiel. English]
    Sandplay : a psychotherapeutic approach to the psyche
/ Dora M. Kalff.
    p. cm.
    Includes bibliographical references and index.
    LCCN 2003104965
    ISBN 0-9728517-0-4

    1. Play therapy. 2. Art therapy. 3. Sandplay--
Therapeutic use. 4. Child psychotherapy.
5. Psychotherapy--Case studies.   I. Title.

RJ505.P6K313 2004   618.92'891653
                           QBI03-200869

Dora M. Kalff

SANDPLAY

A Psychotherapeutic Approach

to the Psyche

TEMENOS PRESS®

Barbara A. Turner, Ph.D., Editor

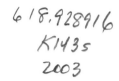

SANDPLAY:
A Psychotherapeutic Approach to the Psyche

©Copyright 2003 Temenos Press®

Published by
TEMENOS PRESS®
Box 305
Cloverdale, California 95425
www.temenospress.com

1 2 3 4 5 6 7 8 9 10

ISBN 0-9728517-0-4

Edited by Barbara A. Turner, Ph.D.
Cover and book design by Charlotte M. Turner, Ph.D.

Original title: Dora M. Kalff, Sandspiel Seine therapeutische Wirkung auf die Psyche
c 1996, 2000 by Ernst Reinhardt Verlag Műnchen Basel
Kemnatenstr. 46, D-80639 Munchen
www.reinhardt-verlag.de

Published in German by Ernst Reinhardt Verlag, ISBN 3-497-01399-4.
Previous English Translation c 1980 by Dora M. Kalff, Sigo Press, ISBN 0-93843400-4.

Printed in the United States of America.

Library of Congress Control Number: 2003104965

Kalff, Dora M.
          Sandplay : a psychotherapeutic approach to the psyche

To my sons and grandson

Peter Baudouin

Martin Michael

Christopher Baudouin

CONTENTS

The Practice of Sandplay Therapy

Advice from Dora Kalff

In the hands of a properly prepared therapist, sandplay is a powerful, invaluable modality. The operative word is "powerful." To the extent that any method can heal, so can it do harm.

Therefore, I urgently advise that even a psychotherapist highly experienced in other methodologies, who contemplates practicing sandplay, should have had a deep personal experience doing a sandplay process as a patient. This should be undertaken with a qualified sandplay therapist. Certified sandplay therapists are members of national sandplay organizations and the International Society for Sandplay Therapy. All sandplay therapists must undertake an extended period of training and careful supervision with a certified sandplay therapist. To attempt to do sandplay in any other way is irresponsible.

NOTE: Information on training in sandplay therapy may be obtained at the Sandplay Therapists of America website,

www.sandplay.org.

PREFACE

We at Temenos Press are honored to bring this new edition of Dora Maria Kalff's *Sandplay: A Psychotherapeutic Approach to the Psyche* to English speaking readers. This book is one of the very few written accounts of the work of Dora Kalff, developer of the Jungian sandplay therapy method. It remains the seminal classic text of sandplay therapy.

By Kalff's simple, yet elegant accounts of actual casework, she presents her theoretical understanding of how psyche and sandplay work. Through her case studies, Kalff invites the reader into her playroom to share an intimate experience of the depths of her connection to her clients and to her work in the sand. In this book, Dora Kalff opens her door, summoning the reader to visit the profoundly transformative possibilities she created with sand, figures, and her presence.

In the editing processes, we have made the sincerest effort to preserve the spirit and intent of Kalff's original German text. In addition, we have earnestly attempted to retain the quality of Kalff's artwork and photographic examples. For historical accuracy, we have maintained the use of the masculine pronoun to conform to the writing style of the time.

Barbara A. Turner, Ph.D.
Editor
2003

SANDPLAY:
A Psychotherapeutic Approach to the Psyche

FOREWORD

Dr. Martin Kalff

I am delighted to introduce the new English translation of *Sandplay: A Psychotherapeutic Approach to the Psyche*, written by my mother, Dora Maria Kalff (1904-1990). As I am working myself with sandplay therapy, I feel grateful for what I have received from my mother. It is also for this reason that I gladly write this foreword and offer my reflections on the method and its roots.

Sandplay is a method of psychotherapy and personal development. This method has three roots, united into a single unit by my mother. Sandplay combines the analytic psychology of C.G. Jung, the World Technique of Margaret Lowenfeld and Eastern thought and philosophy.

It was relatively late in life when my mother took an interest in psychology. She was already 45 years old when she began her six-year course of studies at the C.G. Jung Institute in Zurich. After her divorce in 1949, and the single mother of two sons, three and ten years old, it was necessary that she undertake something new to make a new beginning. Since the war, she lived in a small house in the mountain village of Parpan. As coincidence would have it, the Jung family also spent their vacations in this area. My brother Peter befriended Jung's grandsons. This resulted in what would turn out to be a very crucial meeting between my mother and Carl and Emma Jung. Meeting Carl and Emma Jung inspired Mother to begin analysis and study. The Jungs encouraged her to give serious thought to a method of depth psychology for children. She began her analysis with Emma Jung and worked on special personal issues with C.G. Jung, directly.

My mother came from a sound middle class family that lived in the town of Richterswil on Lake Zurich. She was the next-to-the-youngest child in a family of three girls and one boy. Her father was an influential personality. He owned a textile factory. He was an army colonel and held a high political office corresponding to a congressman in America. At the same time, he had a deep interest in religion and originally would have liked to become a theologian. Her mother was a warm, socially engaged woman, who ran the large household with skill and care.

As a young girl, my mother attended a girls' boarding school in the Engadin. Her Greek teacher inspired her to study Sanskrit and later, basic Chinese. It was here she discovered her interest in Eastern philosophy, Taoism in particular. As a young woman, she was also educated as a concert pianist, studying with Robert Casadesus, who was very well known at the time in Paris. In addition, her studies led her to Italy where she learned the rare craft of bookbinding.

At age 29, she married a Dutch banker and moved to Holland. She and her husband shared a great interest in Asian art. They lived a manorial life with many social obligations and interactions with the royal family. It was into this life that my brother Peter was born in 1939. The fortune of the young family was of short duration however, as difficult times came with the war and the German invasion. German soldiers occupied their house. My mother and little Peter were on the last train out of Holland. She returned alone to Switzerland. A long time of separation from her husband followed, finally resulting in divorce.

So, my mother had already had a diverse life with many difficult experiences when she began her education in psychology. In retrospect, she would say that all of her experiences and the many things she learned had proved important and helpful to her therapeutic work. This applied to her piano studies as well, for she would often include the piano in her work with children.

My mother possessed a great ability to respond to children. C.G. Jung and Emma Jung had originally recognized this quality in her, leading them to encourage her to pursue therapeutic work with children. At the time, however, there were little or no resources for analytic work with children. Analytic work focused on issues of the second half of life and focused on dream work. This type of analysis emphasized verbal communication skills that children have not yet developed. Thus was launched her search for a therapeutic method suitable for children. In 1954 she heard Margaret Lowenfeld speak about her World Technique at a congress in Zurich. A critical feature of this form of therapy was that it gave children the opportunity to express themselves non-verbally with small figurines in a sand box. Margaret Lowenfeld was one of the first therapists to consciously consider the healing aspect of children's pictures as a means of overcoming their disturbances. The tremendous potential of play in overcoming psychic disturbances was greatly underestimated by other therapists.

My mother recognized the great value of this method and decided to study with Lowenfeld at the Institute for Child Psychology, founded in London in 1928. In 1956, she began her yearlong study in London. During this time she also studied with D.W. Winnicott and exchanged professional information with child analyst, M. Fordham.

While doing her work with the World Technique in England, and later in her practice in Zollikon, Switzerland, my mother recognized that the creations of the children in the sand correspond to the inner psychic processes of individuation described by C.G. Jung. She developed her own method for working with these patterns of individuation in the children's work, and in agreement with Margaret Lowenfeld, she called this method *sandplay*.

Mother's first work using sandplay with children proved very effective. It was quite

...my mother recognized that the creations of the children in the sand correspond to the inner psychic processes of individuation described by C.G. Jung. She developed her own method for working with these patterns of individuation in the children's work, and in agreement with Margaret Lowenfeld, she called this method **sandplay**.

by chance that adults began working in sandplay. Parents were astonished at the changes in their children after doing sandplay. Therefore, she proposed that they try it for themselves. By creating their inner images in the sand, remarkable changes also occurred for these people, particularly in the area of their feelings and their outlook on life. It quickly became evident that this non-verbal therapy also provided direct access to the unconscious for adults. It supported in a decisive way positive changes in situations of acute suffering.

The effectiveness of sandplay with adults has been borne out over the years. I hear so many stories of how sandplay has positively changed their lives. Frequently I have heard from former clients of my mother how deeply grateful they are for the experience they had with the sandplay and how this decisively influenced or even saved their lives.

An important aspect of the development of my mother's work was her encounter with eastern spiritual teachers. They brought renewed inspiration and clearly confirmed that profound, archetypal levels of psyche that transcend all cultural boundaries can be touched in sandplay. At the Eranos Conference in 1953-54, Mother met the Japanese Zen Master, Daisetz Suzuki. Suzuki made a great contribution to the Western world by introducing Zen through his writings. Mother visited Suzuki in Japan. Later she had the honor of being the first woman to spend time in a Zen monastery. What impressed her the most about Suzuki was his exquisite ability, and with very simple gestures, to point out that it is precisely in the ordinary, everyday experience that the deepest truths can be illuminated.

She regretted that she was not able to formally study Zen meditation. However, at a later period she received great satisfaction from further conversations with Zen masters, who confirmed that the spirit of Zen is virtually implicit to the sandplay method. This referred not to the outer, formal aspects of the sandplay technique, but to the emphasis on creating a space that awakens and supports the self-healing strengths of the patients. This quality of sandplay resembles an important aspect of Zen, in which the person is thrown back upon him or herself. Both sandplay and Zen emphasize that realization cannot be found in outer authorities, such as teachers or writings, but ultimately only within oneself.

During the time of the Tibetan exile, following the cruel occupation of Tibet by China, Switzerland welcomed 1,000 refugees. Homes for these people were sought with Swiss families. When Mother was asked if she could take on a refugee, she agreed without much hesitation. This was how we came to have a Tibetan monk living with us. Mother gave him a home for eight years. It was through this that she gradually began to have close contact with a variety of Tibetan teachers. We were visited by the teacher of the Dalai Lama, Trichang Rinpoche, and later by the Dalai Lama himself. For Mother this simultaneously awakened an awareness of the rich symbolism of Tibetan Buddhism and a deep compassion for all creatures. This greatly enriched her understanding of the psychic processes of her clients and

...sandplay resembles an important aspect of Zen, in which the person is thrown back upon him or herself. Both sandplay and Zen emphasize that realization cannot be found in outer authorities, such as teachers or writings, but ultimately only within oneself.

worked to further deepen her therapeutic work.

Sandplay soon became internationally known. Mother contributed to this by her ability to communicate effortlessly with colleagues from many countries. Soon she received invitations from interested individuals and institutions around the world. She lectured at clinics, Jung Institutes, and universities, particularly in Italy, Germany, America and Japan. Soon a circle consisting mainly of child analysts and psychologists formed to study the sandplay method. They were earnestly committed to learning and gradually began to use sandplay in their own practices. An especially strong resonance for sandplay developed in the USA and in Japan. Currently, the Japanese Society for Sandplay consists of over one thousand therapists actively practicing sandplay therapy.

SANDPLAY:
A Psychotherapeutic Approach to the Psyche

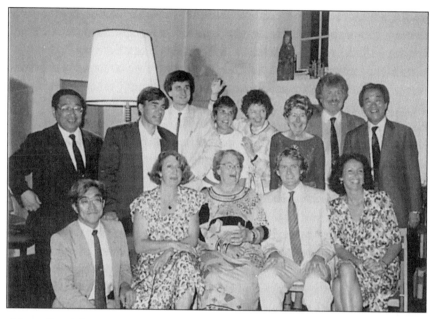

International Society for Sandplay Therapy, Founders Meeting. Zollikon 1985.
Seated Left to Right: Yashuhiro Yamanaka, Andreina Navone, Dora Maria Kalff, Cecil Burney, Paula Carducci. Standing Left to Right: Kazumiko Higuchi, Kaspar Kiepenheuer, Martin Kalff, Chonita Larsen, Estelle Weinrib, Kay Bradway, Joel Ryce-Menuhin, Hayao Kawai.

The non-verbal aspects of sandplay have a particular appeal to the Japanese mind. In Japan, sandplay is known as Hakoniwa Therapy. The name was given to sandplay after the Japanese tradition of making what are known as, hakoniwa, or small, artistic gardens.

After sandplay had gained a foothold in different countries, Mother invited representatives from the various regions to Zollikon for an annual discussion of sandplay work and research. The International Society for Sandplay Therapy, ISST, emerged from this original gathering in 1985. The group included Kay Bradway, Cecil Burney, Chonita Larson and Estelle Weinrib, from America, Paula Carducci and Andreina Navone from Italy, Joel Ryce-Menuhin from England, Professors Higuchi, Kawai, and Yamanaka from Japan, Kaspar Kiepenheuer and myself from Switzerland, and later, in 1986, child analyst, Sigrid Seifert from Germany.

The foundation of the International Society for Sandplay Therapy established statutes for the training and practice of sandplay therapy. Today, ISST facilitates national and international exchange of knowledge and experience with sandplay therapy and provides sandplay education. ISST also maintains an archival library of sandplay cases. Following the foundation of ISST, national and international conferences are held regularly to discuss and exchange information regarding sandplay therapy. There are now three professional sandplay journals. In the USA, there is the Journal of Sandplay Therapy, in Japan, the Archives of Sandplay Therapy, and in Germany, the Magazine of Sandplay Therapy. Sandplay also enjoys a growing body of literature. A detailed bibliography is contained in Mitchell and Friedman's (1994) Sandplay: Past, Present and Future.

As the name implies, *play* is a prominent feature of the sandplay method. The permission to play is built into sandplay therapy. We can say that there is an absence of intentionality inherent to sandplay. In fact, we will often observe that the therapy really gets started at the precise moment the client is able to surrender to the play. This is a highly valuable creative process, because fears, tensions and fixed ideas begin to fall away, quite unintentionally. Deep changes in feeling are activated by the emerging sandplay pictures, when the client's burdens become evident in the sandplay expression. This reflects back upon the client, as in Zen, and sets in motion new hopes that point toward a brighter horizon.

Sandplay creates a bridge between the conscious and the unconscious. During the sandplay process, the conscious mind relaxes its control, allowing penetration to the unconscious material lying beneath the surface. It is important to recognize that the unconscious awakens in the selection of figures and the shaping of the sandplay, and at the same time, the ambitions and purposeful qualities of the conscious mind are silenced. In this way, sandplay promotes what Jung referred to as the transcendent function, making possible a completely new outlook on life. By bringing the conscious and unconscious together in sandplay, significant changes in the conscious attitude toward the unconscious take place. The transformed attitude toward the unconscious facilitates giving the unconscious a voice in times of disturbance. It brings clarity to what might otherwise be unchecked unconscious eruptions, and it fosters the discovery of previously unknown courage and strengths.

Sandplay supports the client's ability to address fears resulting from any number of psychic injuries that have destroyed positive self-development. The deeply disturbing, often psychologically more primitive aspects of the personality can be expressed in sandplay. In this way, these terrifying qualities can be perceived and re-ordered. In the course of sandplay, inner order gradually grows out of chaotic circumstances evidenced early in the work. Sandplay pictures that first express emptiness and loneliness may begin to show new life and growth. Great despair, carefully

The sandplay method takes the limited therapeutic possibilities of language into account with great seriousness and offers alternative means of psychic expression.

hidden behind a façade, can be clearly expressed, and through silent nurture, its destructiveness lessened.

Many of these aspects of the psyche are beyond the limits of ordinary language and cannot be expressed verbally. The sandplay method takes the limited therapeutic possibilities of language into account with great seriousness and offers alternative means of psychic expression. Disturbing life experiences frequently defy expression in words. Witnessing fighting and violence, for example, is highly emotional and confusing. It may only find its full expression in the furious mixing of the sand. What happens in the sandplay is known directly. It is far beyond any number of words the therapist might have.

It is to Margaret Lowenfeld's great credit that she paid attention to the limits of language in therapy. Surely, it was in her work with children that this became evident. However, it is valid for adults as well. Highly articulate adults are at risk of pushing away their real feelings with their facile use of words. As we know, words are very limited in intensely emotional circumstances. Frequently, much more can be said in a non-verbal means of expression. We hardly need convincing that pictures and images are an enormously effective means of moving the psyche, when we consider how we are continually inundated with advertisement and television pictures. It is quite puzzling that we are willing to accept these pictures so passively and hardly make opportunity to actively create our own!

Margaret Lowenfeld perceived great meaning in the pictures she witnessed at her clinic. In her theoretical considerations, she observed expressions of aspects of the psyche that cannot be formulated in words. Lowenfeld called these *proto system*, as she said they are with the child from the beginning of life. She distinguished the proto system from secondary thought processes, specifying that the proto system develops first. Lowenfeld described the proto system as a form of non-verbal thinking. She

characterized it as,

> *...non rational, arranged according to its own laws, extremely personal, idiosyncratic, and by its nature not communicable with words.*

Children express their thinking through their play. Lowenfeld observed that it was critical to healthy development that adequate room be allowed for play. If this is hindered in any way, the proto system energy can remain locked up in the child, prohibiting the investment of any further energy into subsequent tasks of development. This results in apathy and conformity. Lowenfeld observed that as these pre-verbal aspects became visible in the World Technique, the energy contained in them was liberated. Lowenfeld wanted to find a way to understand children's thinking. She wanted a method that would make it possible for the child to express himself or herself in as genuine a way as possible, without the interference of the therapist.

Intending to protect the child from manipulation from the therapist in any way, Lowenfeld greatly emphasized the autonomy of the child and the importance of allowing each child to be who they are. Lowenfeld wanted to exclude the transference of early childhood feelings onto the therapist, as well as the emotional reaction of any counter transference. She received a lot of criticism for doing this. During the course of treatment, she let the children work with a variety of therapists. She emphasized that the transference does not fall on the therapist, but on the sandbox. Rightly so, Lowenfeld recognized the emotional value the sand tray can assume. Recently, more contemporary theoreticians have revised this early observation, emphasizing that it is essential to distinguish three forms of transference, namely: transference onto the contents of the sand tray; transference onto the sand tray itself; and transference through the sand tray in the therapeutic relationship (Montecchi, 1993). As Estelle Weinrib (1983/2003) observed in her book, the sand tray functions in much the same way as Winnicott's transitional object.

The relationship between the client and the therapist assumed new meaning in my mother's work. In contrast to Lowenfeld, she observed that it was the therapist's responsibility to create what she called a free and protected space for the client. She saw that it was in the context of this relationship that the client had the possibility of coming to his or her own deepest center. Mother saw that it was in the safety of this relationship that the client could feel understood. At the same time, in the permission of this relationship the client has the freedom to enter the unknown in his or her play, and in so doing, come to know the Self. In this way the free and protected space may be understood as a *positive transference* in Mother's work. My mother regarded the quality of the relationship as a critical aspect of the client's ability to penetrate to the Self, the deepest layer of the psyche, according to C.G. Jung. In order for this experience to occur in therapy, it is certainly necessary that the therapist, through their own continued work, develop a living relationship to their own wholeness.

I am very pleased that *Sandplay: A Psychotherapeutic Approach to the Psyche* is being reissued in America. America figured prominently in the development of Mother's work. Her ideas were received there with particular openness and enthusiasm. Actually, I observed that she was energetic and joyful when she returned from her frequent visits to the States. One would never think that she was returning from such an intense schedule of lectures, workshops. and countless individual sessions! This support provided her great energy to further cultivate and deepen this important tool for psychotherapy and inner development.

Happily, we now have a growing body of literature on sandplay. Nonetheless, this classical text remains fundamental to the understanding and study of sandplay therapy. Perhaps even better than a more technical text, its simple manner of telling the stories of the therapy sessions captures the underlying flavor and attitude of the way my mother worked.

March 2003

Dr. Martin Kalff
Zollikon, Switzerland

NOTES

Lowenfeld, M. (1979/1993). *Understanding Children's Sandplay: Lowenfeld's World Technique*. Cambridge: Margaret Lowenfeld Trust.

Mitchell, R.R. & Friedman, H. (1994). *Sandplay: Past, Present and Future*. London: Routledge.

Montecchi, F. (1993). *Giocando con la sabbia: La psichoterapia con bambini e adolescenti et la sandplay therapy*. Franco Angelli.

Weinrib, Estelle L.(1983/2003) *Images of the self: The sandplay therapy process*. Cloverdale, CA: Temenos Press.

Archives of Sandplay Therapy. Edited and published by: The Japan Association of Sandplay Therapy.

Journal of Sandplay Therapy. Sandplay Therapists of America.

Magazine for Sandplay-therapy. Publishing house sandplay-therapy, Landauerstr. Vol. 16, D-14197 Berlin, Germany. (pp. 166)

CHAPTER 1

SANDPLAY:
A Pathway to the Psyche

In my sandplay work with children and adolescents, I have observed evidence of the individuation process, as described by C.G. Jung. In the material that follows, I would like to illustrate these findings with several case stories of development that occurred in my playroom. First, however, a few clarifications are necessary.

My observations agree with Jung's theory that that the Self directs the process of psychic development from the time of birth. The *Self*, according to Jung, "...designates the whole range of psychic phenomena in man. It expresses the unity of the personality as a whole." The Self consists of both the conscious and unconscious components of the psyche.[1] Man is born as a totality which, according to Erich Neumann, is kept preserved for the time being within the mother's Self.[2] When all of the requirements of the newborn infant, such as appeasement of hunger, shelter from cold, etc., are met by the bodily mother, the child experiences an unconditional security and a sense of safety through motherly love. We call this first phase the *mother-child unity*.

After one year, the Self of the child--the center of his psychic totality--separates itself from the Self of the mother. In the second phase, the child experiences more and more security in the relationship to the mother through her caresses and displays of tenderness. A relationship of trust grows out of this experience.

(The security that results from this primary relationship is the basis of the third phase. (During this phase, which begins around the end of the second year of life and at the beginning of the third, the center of the Self is stabilized in the unconscious of the child and begins to manifest itself in symbols of wholeness.) (During this time the child plays, draws, paints or speaks in symbols of wholeness.) The child uses the same ancient language of symbols that adult man has used, consciously or unconsciously, to express his wholeness throughout the ages and in all cultures. These symbols are either human figures of godly content, like the figures of Christ, Mary, Buddha, etc., or they are of a geometric or numerical nature, such as the circle or the square. We accept the validity of these symbols of the wholeness of the human psyche, because they have occurred everywhere without exception from the earliest times of man. Jung observed that the circle, particularly as a symbol of perfection and of perfect being, is a well-known expression of God, of heaven, the sun, the soul, and of the ideal of man **[Illustrations 1, 2, 3 and 4]**. The square, my experience has shown, appears when wholeness is developing.

I have observed that in psychic development, the entity of four appears either before the symbol of the circle or in connec-

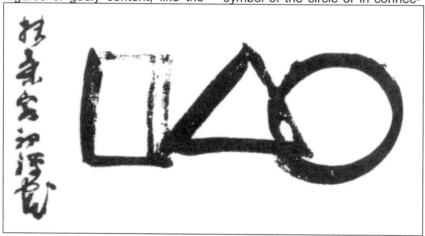

Illustration 1: Geometric shapes as an image of totality. Brush and Ink. *The World of Zen.* Sengai.

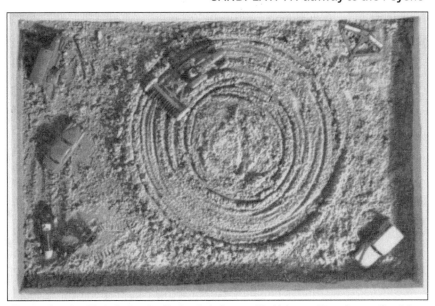

Illustration 2: *Circle in Sand.* Circle of wholeness tilled into sand by a farmer. Sandplay. Eleven-year-old boy.

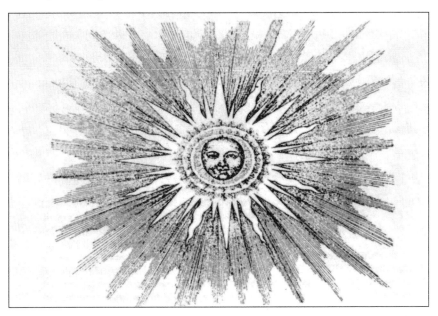

Illustration 3: Circular sun as an image of perfect being. *Symbols of Transformation.* Jung.

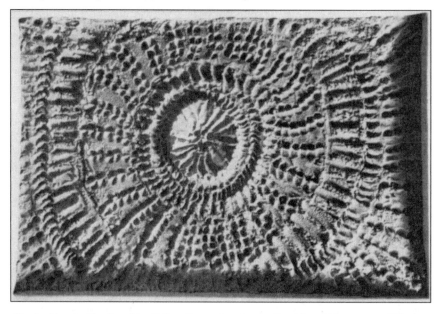

Illustration 4: *The Sun*. The Self as the centered sun. Sandplay. Fifteen-year-old boy.

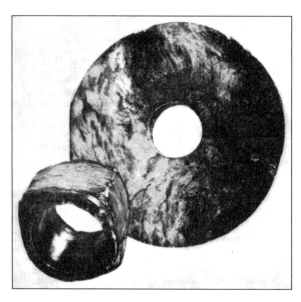

Illustration 5: Heaven as round and earth as square. Sculpture. Chou Dynasty, China. *Chinese Art.*, MacKenzie.[3]

tion with the circle **[Illustrations 5, 6 and 7]**.

My ideas were confirmed a few years ago in San Francisco when I saw Rhoda Kellogg's collection of children's artwork. During her many years as director of a nursery school, she collected thousands of drawings and finger paintings by children from two to four years of age.

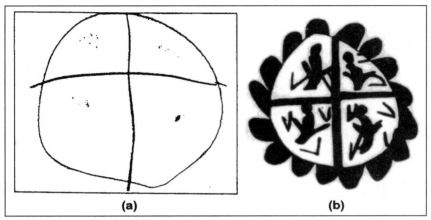

(a)	**(b)**

Illustration 6: (a) Emergent image of psychic wholeness as circle and squares. Drawing. Three-year-old child. (b) More evolved image of Self with budding human forms. Painting. Six-year-old child. *Analyzing Children's Art.* Kellogg.[4] (Kellogg graphics reproduced with permission from The McGraw Hill Companies.)

An enormous number of these pictures showed the familiar well-known symbols of wholeness.

Such symbols appear not only in drawings and paintings of children, but also in their verbal communication. A three-year-old boy asked me one day, "If it is true that the earth is round and that God can see everybody, does that mean He is like a circle?" Over each of his

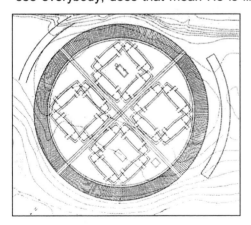

drawings, on the upper side of the picture, he drew a blue line from one end to the other. When I asked what the lines meant, he answered that it was God. These lines, each a very small part of an enormous circle, told of his conception.

Another boy of about the same age once discovered some tin figures on my piano. He positioned them to form a full circle. He left the room for a while, and when

Illustration 7: Early Viking village shaped as squares in quartered circle. Diagram of Danish excavation. Danish National Museum.

5

he came back, he brought a small, white porcelain dove and put it behind a photograph that was on the piano. When I asked him what the dove was doing in this hiding place, he answered, "We can't see God either."

Through such statements from children we can see the numinous content of the symbol. The circle is not only a geometrical form; it is also a symbol that brings to light something which lives invisibly in man. Symbols speak for the inner, energy-laden pictures of the innate potentials of the human being which, when they are manifested, continue to influence the development of man. These symbols of numinous or religious content tell of an inner drive for spiritual order that allows relationship to the deity. This spiritual order gives man an inner security and insures for him, among other things, the development of his inherent personality.

I want to emphasize that the manifestation of the Self, this inner order, this pattern of wholeness, is the most important moment in the development of the personality. Psychotherapeutic work has proven that healthy development of the ego can take place only as a result of the successful manifestation of the Self. The Self may manifest as a dream symbol or as a depiction in the sandbox. Such a manifestation of the Self seems to guarantee the development and consolidation of the personality.

Symbols speak for the inner, energy-laden pictures of the innate potentials of the human being which, when they are manifested, continue to influence the development of man.

On the other hand, in the case of weak or neurotic ego development, I assume with certainty that the manifestation of the Self through symbol has failed to appear. This may happen because the necessary motherly protection has not been given, or because the Self manifestation has been critically disturbed by external influences such as war, illness, or lack of understanding from the environment during the child's early development. Therefore, I aim to give the child's Self the possibility of constellating and manifesting in therapy. Through the transference I try to protect it and to stabilize the relationship between the Self and the ego. This is possible within the psychotherapeutic relationship because it corresponds to the natural tendency of the psyche to constellate itself when a free and sheltered space is created. This free space occurs in the therapeutic setting when the therapist is fully able to accept the child so that the therapist, as a person, is as much a part of everything going on in the room as is the child himself. When a child feels that he is not alone, not only in his distress but also in his happiness, he then feels free and protected in all his expressions. This relationship of confidence is of great importance, for in some instances, the first phase of psychic development, the mother-child unity, can be restored. This psychic situation can establish an inner peace that contains the potential for development of the total personality. This includes its intellectual and spiritual aspects.

It is the role of the therapist to perceive these possibilities and, like the guardian of a precious treasure, protect them in their development. For the child,

the therapist represents the protector, the space, the freedom and at the same time, the boundaries. The unique occurrence of each phase of development is of great consequence, because the transformations of psychic energy necessary for the individual can occur only within these parameters.

Gerhard Tersteegen, a 17th-Century mystic and pastor, lived by the following principle: "Whoever deals with souls must be like a nursemaid who leads the child by a halter and who only protects it from dangers and falls, but otherwise must allow the child to go its own way." It seems to me that he was saying that no unambiguous theories exist for the cure of souls. One must recognize the uniqueness of each person so that with the help of wise guidance, free development of individuality can be assured.

Development under the care of a therapist can be compared to the goal set by Pestalozzi in his work on education, *How Gertrud Teaches Her Children*. Pestalozzi said that it is through genuine love by the mother that the child finds his way to inner unity and thus gains access to the divine.[5]

According to my experi-

7

ence, a healthy ego can develop only in the condition of the child's total security. In the case of a weak ego I must assume that the manifestation of the Self as a symbol, which is normally observed between the ages of two to three years, has not taken place. Amazingly enough, I have found that where the symbolic manifestation of the Self was not made possible during childhood, it can often be recovered to a certain degree in therapy. This recovery can occur at any stage of life.

Jung himself says:

> In my experience it is of considerable practical importance that the symbols aiming at wholeness should be correctly understood by the doctor. They are the remedy with whose help neurotic dissociations can be repaired, by restoring to the conscious mind a spirit and an attitude which from time immemorial have been felt as solving and healing in their effects. They are *ré-presentations collectives* which facilitate the much-needed union of conscious and unconscious. This union cannot be accomplished either intellectually or in a purely practical sense, because in the former case the instincts rebel and in the latter case reason and morality. Every dissociation that falls within the category of the psychogenic neuroses is due to a conflict of this kind, and the conflict can only be resolved through the symbol.[6]

In this sense, we can also understand Bachofen when he writes: "That is precisely the great dignity of the symbol, that it allows, and even stimulates, different degrees of comprehension, and leads from the truths of the physical life to those of a higher spiritual order."[7] The symbol embodies the image of a psychic content that transcends consciousness and points to the eternal foundation of our nature given us by God. Once recognized and experienced, it leads man to the authentic dignity of his existence as a human being.

The symbol plays a great role in sandplay therapy, which I have expanded from the Lowenfeld World Technique.[8] I use a sand box with dimensions 28.5 x 19.5 x 3 inches. This size confines the player's imagination and thus acts as a regulating, protecting factor.

Hundreds of small figures of every conceivable type are provided. The child arranges any figures he chooses in the sand. The sand picture that is produced by the child can be understood as a three-dimensional representation of some aspect of his psychic situation. An unconscious problem is played out in the sand box, just like a drama. The conflict is transferred from the inner world to the outer world and is made visible. This game of fantasy influences the dynamics of the unconscious in the child and thus moves his psyche.

The analyst interprets for himself the symbols emerging in the course of a series of sand pictures. The therapist's understanding of the problem that emerges in the picture often promotes an atmosphere of trust between the analyst and the child. This trust is like the original mother-child unity and exerts a healing influence. It is not necessary to communicate the therapist's insights to the child in words, as we are dealing with the experience of the symbol in the free and sheltered space. Under certain circumstances however, the pictures are interpreted to the child in an easily understandable way that is connected with his life

situation. With the help of the exterior picture, the inner problem becomes visible and brings about the next step in development. In this process, new energies are freed that lead to the formation of healthy ego development.

In addition, the details and composition of the pictures give the therapist an indication of the path to follow in the treatment. Frequently the initial picture gives information about the situation. Hidden in the symbols it may contain the path to the goal of the realization of the Self. An eight-year-old boy has represented the normal development of these energies very nicely in a sand picture [Illustration 8]. In the upper right side of the picture the Self is embodied in the good shepherd with the sheep. Dark foreign powers (Moroccans) in orderly rows move toward the space that can be regarded as representing the boy's inner peace. The powers are armed. The boy remarked, however, "Actually they wouldn't need to be armed," sensing he could cope with them. My experience in sandplay coincides with Erich Neumann's theory of the stages of ego-development.[9] These are: 1) the animal, vegetative stage; 2) the fighting stage; and 3) the adaptation to the col-

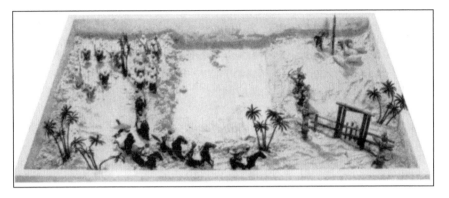

Illustration 8: Dark, unconscious energies move in an orderly fashion toward the Self. Sandplay. Eight-year-old boy.

lective. In the first phase, the ego expresses itself chiefly in pictures where animals and vegetation predominate. The next stage brings battles that appear again and again, especially during puberty. By now, the child is so strengthened that he can take upon himself the battle with external influences and is able to come to grips with them. Finally, he is admitted to the environment as a person and becomes a member of the collective.

While studying Chinese thought, I came across a diagram that seems to correspond to our viewpoint [**Illustration 9**]. It is the diagram of Chou Tun Yi, a philosopher of the Sung period, who lived around the year 1000 ce. The beginning of all things is

Phases of Psychic Development

BIRTH

1. **Mother-Child Unity**
2. **Relationship of Child to Mother**
3. **Constellation of the Self**
4. **Ego Development (Neumann)**
   a) **Animal Vegetative**
   b) **Battle**
   c) **Integration into the Collective**

shown in a circle, in which I see an analogy to the Self at birth. A second circle shows the interfusing action of yin and yang that produces the five elements. I am inclined to relate this circle to what I have said about the manifestation of the Self. It contains the germ of those energies that lead to the formation of the ego

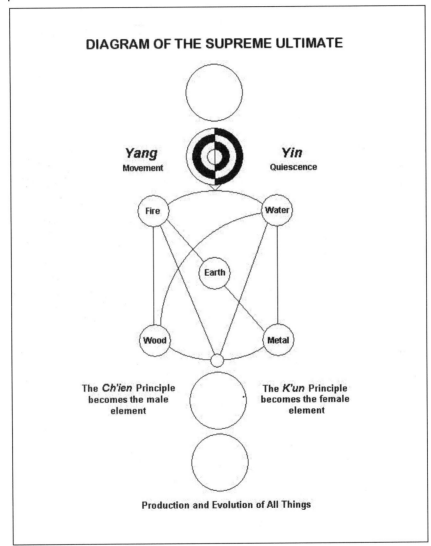

DIAGRAM OF THE SUPREME ULTIMATE

Yang
Movement

Yin
Quiescence

Fire

Water

Earth

Wood

Metal

The *Ch'ien* Principle
becomes the male
element

The *K'un* Principle
becomes the female
element

Production and Evolution of All Things

Illustration 9: Graphic representation of developmental progression of body and psyche. Chou Tun Yi, Chinese Philosopher 1000 ce.

and the development of personality **[Illustrations 10 and 11]**. Just as the five elements arise from this constellation, the personality develops around the centering point of the ego. I equate this step with development in the first half of life. Also, in our tradition, five is the number of the natural man **[Illustrations 12 and 13]**. Here, man is pictured as a pentagram with his head and outstretched arms and legs. He is a microcosm in the macrocosm. The third circle could be compared with the manifesta-

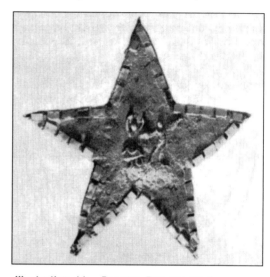

Illustration 11: *Dancers.* Boy and girl dance on a five pointed star. Masculine and feminine energies interact on symbol of the whole person. Plaster sculpture. Twelve-year-old girl.

tion of the Self in the individuation process during the second half of life. In the fourth circle, I see the ending as opposed to the beginning. Here I see the end of the movement that leads from life to death. Following the law of transformation, on which the diagram is based, death, just like the sacrifice of a psychic situation lived to its conclusion, holds the germ of new life.

These images may show us that in all traditions, our lives cor-

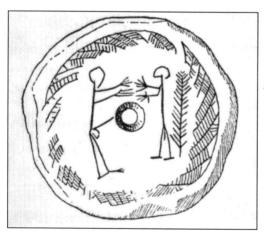

Illustration 10: Man and woman enter embrace in centered circle. The germ of the ego formed by the interaction of opposites emerging from the Self. Drawing on bone. Denmark.

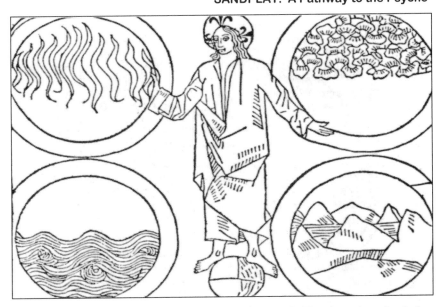

Illustration 12: Christ, as totality, stands on globe of earth. The elements earth, air, fire and water pour into the four spherical quadrants of the material world. *Psychology and Alchemy*. Jung.

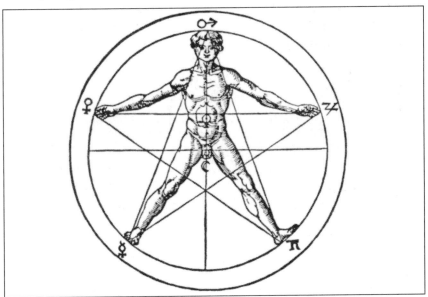

Illustration 13: Man as microcosm in five pointed star. Tyco Brahe, *Calendarium Naturale Magicum Perpetuum* (1582).

respond to a physical and psychic flow that can be looked on as the basis of individual development. Therefore, it seems to me that our therapeutic efforts with the child and adolescent will do justice only as seen from this view.

The children who come to me for treatment suffer mostly from lack of inner security. They have no feeling of belonging. Something prevents the normal growth that is necessary for their inner balance. This may be an unfavorable home or a situation outside the home. Because of this, I believe that it is very important not to separate the place of my practice from the environment and atmosphere of my home. [Illustrations 14a and 14b]. When my heavy entrance door closes (my house was first constructed in 1485), the child enters an old, paneled room in which a magnificent tile stove is quite prominent. It is easy to climb a few built-in steps leading to the top of the stove. The child can now do what he feels like doing. He is allowed to sit or lie on the stove. He can look down on the room or out through the window, where he can watch the birds that play and bathe in the little fountain in my garden. He can look at some picture books or read magazines. He may also feel encouraged to investigate the unusual objects and pictures in my old house. My home's irregular order of rooms and staircases heightens its interest. Small children often love to play hide-and-seek, while the older ones sometimes become adventurous and look for hidden treasures. If possible, I give them free range of the house. Often I take them to the basement, where they investigate the meter-thick walls to see if there are subterranean passages. We may go to the immense attic, with its secret double floors that invite them to explore. The children are always looking for something hidden, a treasure which they would like to find in themselves that they have so far been unable to discover.

My house was constructed hundreds of years ago on rock. Its rooms were not built and shaped with a yardstick and compass, but grew according to a natural law. This house offers an atmosphere that corresponds to the natural temperament of young people. Moreover, the child comes upon a world that is completely open to him, and where he is totally welcomed and accepted. As he enters the playroom where the sand tray is waiting, the chain

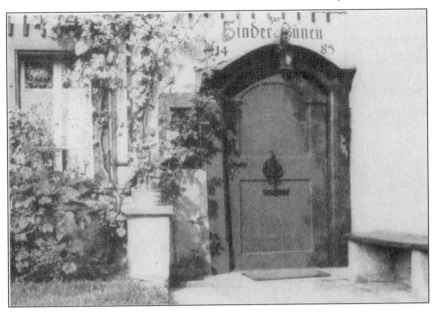

Illustration 14a: Entrance door to Kalff house, *Hinder Zünen 8.* Built 1485.

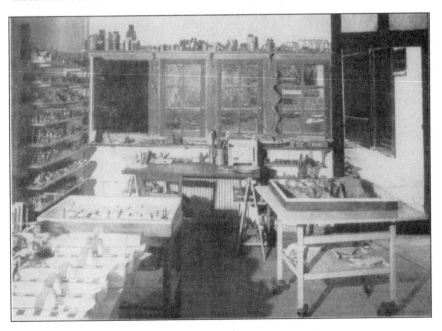

Illustration 14b: Dora Kalff's playroom.

of tension that perhaps arose by wondering, "What will I find, what will I have to do?" is broken.

There are many things in my playroom: paints, clay, mosaic, plaster of Paris, etc. They lie invitingly open on a large table. The sand trays are close by and on a shelf are hundreds of little figures made of lead and other materials. There are people, not only of various types and professions of modern times, but also figures from past centuries. There wild and domestic animals, houses of different styles, trees, bushes, flowers, fences, traffic signals, cars, trains, old carriages and boats. In short, everything that exists in the world, as well as in fantasy, is made available.

All of the items listed above are the materials that Dr. Lowenfeld collected for her World Play.[10] She understood how to place herself in the world of the child. With ingenious intuition she created a game that enables the child to build a world, his world, in a sand box. [Illustrations 15a and 15b]. The size of the box corresponds exactly to what the eye can encompass. From among the numerous objects, the child chooses those that particularly appeal to him and are meaningful.

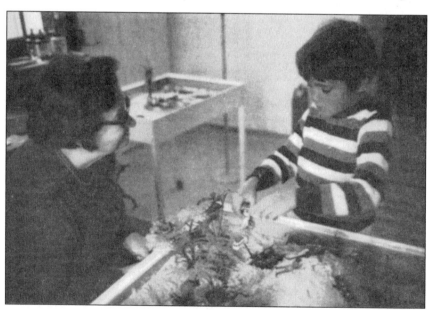

Illustration 15a: Dora Kalff engaged in sandplay with young child.

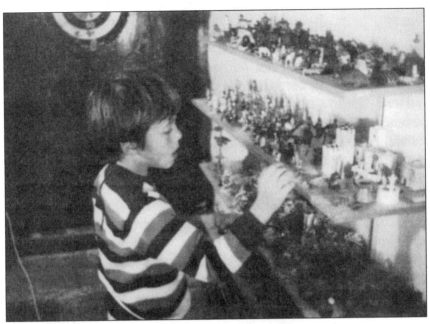

Illustration 15b: Child considers figures for his sandplay.

He forms hills, tunnels, plains, lakes and rivers in the sand in the same way he views the world from his own situation. He allows the figures to act as he experiences them in his fantasy. The child has absolute freedom in determining what to construct, which figures to choose and how to use them. The same limitations that are prerequisite for genuine freedom in the real world are present in the measurements of the sandbox. They are scaled down to one-person size, thereby forming limits to what can be represented and providing a frame wherein transformation can take place. Quite unconsciously, the child experiences what I call a free, and at the same time, protected space.

Using several cases, I will try to illustrate the experience that occurs within this space. In order to protect the patients, I have had to omit certain information.

SANDPLAY:
A Psychotherapeutic Approach to the Psyche

NOTES

1. C. G. Jung, *Symbols of Transformation*, Vol. 5, Collected Works. (New York: Pantheon Books, Inc., 1967).

2. E. Neumann, *The Child*. (New York: G. P. Putnam's Sons, 1973).

3. F. MacKenzie, *Chinese Art*. (New York: Marboro Books, 1961).

4. R. Kellogg, *Analyzing Children's Art*. (National Press Books, Palo Alto, CA, 1970).

5. J. H. Pestalozzi, *Wie Gertrud ihre Kinder lehrt*, in Jung's Collected Works, Vol. 9. (Zurich: Racher, 1945).

6. C. G. Jung, *Psychology and Religion, General Remarks on Symbolism*, Vol. 11, Collected Works. (New York: Pantheon Books, Inc., 1963),191.

7. J. J. Bachofen, *Mutlerrecht and Urreligion* (Leipzig: Kroner, 1926).

8. R. Bowyer, *Lowenfeld World Technique: Studies in personality*. (New York: Pergamon Press, Inc., 1970).

9. Neumann.

10. M. Lowenfeld, *The Non-verbal Thinking of Children and its Place in Psychology*. (London: The Institute of Child Psychology, 1964).

CHAPTER 2

CHRISTOPH:
Anxiety
9-Year-Old Boy

Nine-year-old Christoph came to my house led by his father, a tall, robust farmer. The boy gave the impression of being overly delicate and anxious. At my request, he willingly followed me into the playroom. Hesitating, yet curious, he looked around. Small curls framed his pale forehead. I wondered how such a fragile boy could be from the rugged countryside. After a while his glance fell on the small cap pistol, which was situated at some distance from him. "Would you like to play with it?" I asked him. A slight, but definite defensive movement told me that he was afraid of the pistol.

I learned from his father that the school authorities had requested that Christoph see a psychologist because he frequently played truant. Each day the boy left his house punctually for school and returned home at the expected time. His mother, therefore, had no idea that there were many times when he had not gone to school. Christoph lived with his parents and a brother, who was two years younger, in fairly isolated, rural surroundings. On his way to the village school, he passed through meadows with fruit trees. What he might have done while the other children were in school, no one knew.

Christoph glanced at the sand tray. "Have you ever played with sand?" I asked.

"Yes, I used to," he answered, "...but now that's only for my little brother. I'm too big for that."

"But I bet you haven't played in sand with toys and figures like these." I showed him my collection. That appealed to him, and he quickly set to work. In the middle of the sand tray appeared a large hill. With great care he hollowed out a tunnel. He was satisfied only when he could see straight through it. Then he turned to the figures. A small house seemed to please him, and he placed it in the lower left corner. Next to it he put a swing. He fenced these in without making an opening for entering or leaving. On the top of the hill he planted a tall poplar tree. Beneath it, under its shelter, he positioned a small child on a bench. A narrow path led from the mound to the plain below **[Illustration 16]**.

Suddenly he became lively and selected heavy tanks, soldiers and weapons. He placed them around and all over the hill. "A war has broken out," he said. Soldiers besieged the hill, machine gunners shot through the tunnel, and the tanks were prepared for combat. He even wanted a bomber plane hung from the ceiling by a thread, so the hill could be attacked from the

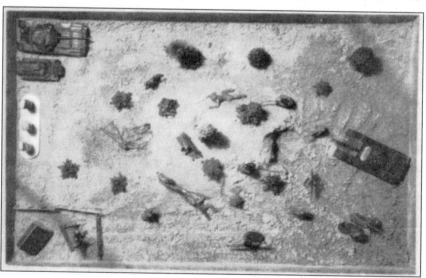

Illustration 16: Forces in the outer world threaten the development of the little boy who sits atop the rounded hill. The shade tree and the filling station hold the potential for overcoming his great fears.

air. This boy, who had been so shy and worried at the beginning of the hour, now seemed to be gripped by a passion to make certain that everything was exactly the way he wanted. Christoph looked at his picture with satisfaction and made sure that the bomber would not miss its target. Before leaving the room, he suddenly put a filling station on the left edge of the picture. His face was aglow as he went to meet his father, whom he asked to look at what he had done.

On the one hand, the picture showed a peaceful situation—the way it might be at his home: a house, a small garden and a small boy on a swing. Here, he seemed to feel at ease. At the same time, up on the hill near a tall poplar tree, there sat another boy with whom Christoph identified as well.

The tree has preoccupied man from time immemorial. It is rooted deeply in the nourishing earth. Its trunk grows up toward the sky and its branches unfold into a crown that blooms in spring and carries fruit in autumn. Its growth can be compared to man's life. In many cultures it is represented as the tree of life. Men seek protection in its shade. Its fruit appeases hunger and quenches thirst. In this way, the tree embodies both protecting and nourishing elements.

The boy dreamed up there on the hilltop. In the shelter of the tree he longed to develop the talents that would allow him to take his proper place in the world. At the same time the war raged around the hill, threatening this wish. The outside world seemed to him an unconquerable opponent. Anxiously, he withdrew into his temenos, the fenced-in, sheltered space of his house.

As I looked at his hill, I was reminded involuntarily of the shape of a pregnant woman's abdomen. I wondered why of all things, this hill would be the target of those attacks. Could it be that his mother had gone through an

The outside world seemed to him an unconquerable opponent. Anxiously, he withdrew into his temenos, the fenced-in, sheltered space of his house.

unfortunate pregnancy? Was the boy's search for other feminine protection than that provided by his own mother that drove him to the situation under the tree on the hill? I concluded that a discussion with his mother might provide some information.

Christoph's mother told me that she grew up on a poor farm and had a difficult life. Often she did not feel well and suffered from abdominal pains. However little attention was paid to this. Instead she was scolded for being lazy when she felt ill. The pains continued even after she married. She feared becoming pregnant, and she needed reassurance from several doctors that there was nothing to worry about in giving birth to a child. As soon as she became pregnant, fear of the delivery became almost unbearable. Again, she needed the constant reassurance of a doctor. Finally, she was able to wait patiently for the birth. She had a normal delivery. However, she had hardly begun to take on the responsibility for the infant, when she was plagued with new fears.

We might assume, therefore, the boy never really found a feeling of security with his mother. It is even possible to perceive that the fears of the mother were transferred to the child.

In addition, little Christoph had experienced a great many unfortunate episodes in his younger life. When he was barely two years old he stuck his finger in a wall socket and received an electric shock. Before he started school he was operated on for a hernia. This also seems to have persistently intimidated him. His mother told me that he was very frightened of injections and doctors in white coats. He was afraid of the dark, and at night he feared going upstairs alone in his room.

During his second year in school, he had a teacher who handled the children roughly. This increased his anxiety and may have led eventually to his staying away from school. At this point he also began to steal small objects from his mother, especially candy.

As a first step it became necessary to provide the boy the security that would enable him to face the difficulties in life.

In his picture he had shown that he was looking for a safe place outside his home. He saw himself on top of the hill being sheltered by the tree, since he was seeking a symbolic mother. On the other hand, the tree is also a symbol of the Self. It embodies not only maternal femininity, but its straight trunk also has a phallic meaning. Thus, it is a carrier of the union of opposites. From a prognostic point of view, I had hope that a centering of the natural energies within the boy was possible. I was also pleased that Christoph put a filling station at the left edge of the picture at the last minute. This indicated that new energies could spring from the unconscious!

By the second session Christoph seemed to be completely at ease with me. He decided which game to play. At first a small store was the greatest attraction. He wanted to come to it and buy things from me. There were fruits of all kinds, groceries and candy. He bought large quantities of oranges. No wonder, since the shining sphere contained a sweet, juicy fruit and seeds that symbolized new life. This was what the boy's unconscious was striving to attain.

In spite of his wish to be permitted to use the large surface, I was surprised when he painted a tiny man in the bottom corner. Yes, that was still the size of his small ego!

In another session the peaceful store game came to an abrupt end when Christoph suddenly staged a raid on the shop. He was the attacker and he made me the policeman who had to look for him. Christoph had great fun hiding in the secret places of our old house, which meant I had to search for him a long time. Often, I prolonged the search on purpose to show him how well he had hidden himself. Wasn't this game showing how Christoph wanted me to uncover his own inner secrets? He wanted to be taken seriously. He wanted to be searched for.

Later he revealed that he, just like his father, was fond of drawing. He wanted to draw on the large white board (2.50 x 1m). In spite of his wish to be permitted to use the large surface, I was surprised when he painted a tiny man in the bottom corner. Yes, that was still the size of his small ego!

After a month he made a second sand picture. Again, a boy sat on a hill with a small village spread out below. Ducks and geese walked about on the village square. Suddenly he changed the peaceful village into a battleground by placing fighting soldiers throughout. Cars and a train were stuck in the hill. This picture demonstrated that hardly any progress had been achieved in the preceding month.

Nevertheless, Christoph became bolder and bolder. He even became interested in the cap pistol. He wanted to know what could be done with it. First I showed him how to hold it so that the trigger could be squeezed. Finally, he wanted to hear the noise. He wanted me to shoot while he stood far away and put his fingers in his ears. Two or three times he watched and listened. Then he wanted to make it work himself. He wanted it louder and louder. Eventually we ended up in the cellar, where he exploded countless detonator caps on the stone floor. I could not supply him with enough caps. The louder the noise, the happier he became.

About four months went by before he made another sand picture. With his hands he drew broad streets in the sand and put some cars moving about. In contrast to his first pictures, this one appeared empty and meaningless. However, it was the first time that no obstacles were placed in the road. The cars could circulate freely. The damned-up libido was beginning to flow! I hoped that it would not take long for a definite step forward to be seen in his life.

In the next hour, he again drew on the large white board. This time, he filled almost all the available space. The picture represented a ski race. Many people lined the ski track to watch a skier who was dashing downhill. This picture confirmed my impression that the energy that had been held back in his unconscious was being activated. It was now in motion and trying to move toward a goal. The outer world where fighting soldiers had at first represented obstacles to his development, had now changed into a crowd that watched and admired the achiever, the skier. It was very clear to me that considerable ambition lay hidden in this seemingly delicate child.

It was too soon to assume that Christoph was capable of handling this energy, but I was delighted to perceive that the healing influence of the psyche had begun to come through. The drawing hinted at the child's potential; however, its weak strokes clearly indicated to me what the next step was. Its realization was still in the future. From my past observations, I know that a minimum of six to eight weeks is needed before a situation that is just becoming visible as it emerges from the unconscious can push through into outer life. It is as delicate as a newly sprouting blade of grass that needs attentive care. With increased confidence I looked forward to Christoph's next session.

He came a week later, but the expression on his face worried me. He was paler than ever and he looked around anxiously. What could have happened? I greeted him with the question, "How are you?"

"Not well," he answered. "I've just seen an accident." Christoph had to take a short train ride to come to see me. He had seen a postman, who was bringing packages to the tram, fall from his wagon as the train began to move. The man was not hurt at all, however, the few seconds of uncertainty before Christoph knew whether the postman was badly hurt or not were enough to destroy the security that was just beginning to build within him.

From my past observations, I know that a minimum of six to eight weeks is needed before a situation that is just becoming visible as it emerges from the unconscious can push through into outer life.

This was all clearly expressed in the sand picture that he made while still suffering from the effects of the accident **[Illustration 17]**. He put the figures in the sand totally at random. Tanks, soldiers, domesticated animals, as well as those from the steppes and the jungle, filled the sandbox to the rim without grouping or design. A train was stuck in the sand. The representation reminded me of pictures made by schizophrenic patients. In my concern over this big setback that the boy suffered, I tried to look for some positive elements. On the lower left side was a small pond. In front near a large blossoming tree sat a small boy

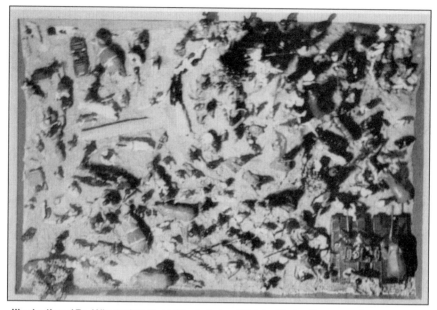

Illustration 17: Witnessing an accident shakes Christoph's fragile sense of security. The flowering tree and the pond from which an elephant drinks are hopeful indicators in this chaotic presentation.

and a woman with their backs to the chaos. An elephant was the only animal turning toward the pond to drink water. Christoph added, "I wouldn't like to live in a world like that." He sought refuge in the therapeutic situation that he represented by the child and woman. He already had the experience that security could be found here. He also knew that he gained new strength from unknown sources (his own unconscious, symbolized by the water). In addition, the tree in bloom represents the Self that directs the growth process. The elephant that can be seen as belonging to

a group, probably stood for the high demands the boy carried in himself.

Animals represent various aspects of human instincts, and it is therefore important that we consider their significance. The elephant possesses a high degree of intelligence and helps man with his work in the jungle. In India, the elephant is holy because it is a legendary creator of Buddha. Therefore, the elephant embodies, among other things, the preconscious animal form of the Redeemer.

By saying that he did not

want to live in that kind of world, Christoph expressed his hope for the redemption that he unconsciously and symbolically revealed in the small group around the pond. Of course, the overwhelming force of the chaotic situation that surrounded him still seemed much too powerful.

At that point in time, Christoph's teacher established contact with me. I was gratified to learn from him that the boy was no longer skipping school. However, he was having great difficulty in keeping up with his classmates in his studies. The teacher suggested that Christoph be transferred to a special class. I was afraid that this might cause a new shock for the boy. His ambition, which still slumbered in his unconscious, but showed up so strongly in his pictures, would be hurt. The little security that Christoph had gained might be destroyed again.

I asked the teacher to be patient and, if at all possible, to keep Christoph in the class. It seemed crucial at this time to give Christoph every opportunity to become psychically stronger. The fragile improvements that he worked so hard to achieve needed to be preserved.

In therapy, more ways had to be found which could restore Christoph's shaky trust in himself.

When he came for the next hour, he discovered a broken-down electric locomotive. He wanted to take it apart, find out why it wouldn't work and repair it. Even older boys had tried to do the same without success. Nevertheless I let him do as he pleased. He took great pains loosening the small screws and tiny parts and laid them in precise order on the table in front of him. I admired his manual dexterity and the care with which he handled even the tiniest pieces. By the end of the hour they all lay neatly in rows. Would it be possible for Christoph to put them back together in the right order? He asked me to leave the parts just as he had placed them.

In the two succeeding hours Christoph sat at the table intensely occupied with reconstructing the small locomotive. From time to time, he tried it out. When it did not function, he would again change something. Suddenly it began to move. What a surprise! What joy! He quickly constructed a train track on the floor.

After that many hours passed with both of us on the

floor, while he instructed me about throwing switches and stopping trains. Because I am not very good in these matters, anyway, I let him direct me. He obviously enjoyed this. If I forgot something, such as throwing a switch, it gave him the chance to correct me. He became my teacher in this game and thus grew into a new role. Here, he knew something that I still had to learn!

After five weeks of intense playing, I suggested a sand picture, and Christoph quickly agreed **[Illustration 18]**. A wide bridge leading out of a forest spans a river on which boats cruise in both directions. On the bridge itself is heavy traffic. A train and some cars rush back and forth.

Many forces and new energies had been set in motion and were emerging from the unconscious, represented by the forest. By looking more closely, I noticed that some of the vehicles had definite regulating functions. For instance, a fire engine rushes to put out flames and the garbage truck collects the trash. Regulatory energies now moved to resolve the chaotic condition of the

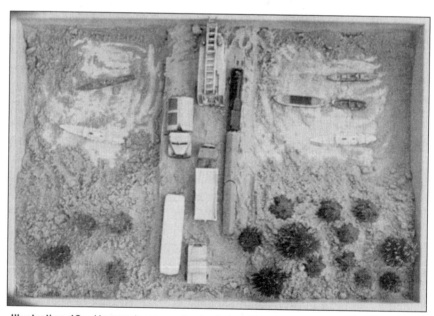

Illustration 18: Unconscious energies begin to move along channeled, regulated pathways in all four directions, as the shape of the square emerges in the sandplay.

preceding picture. The traffic circulates in both directions, on the water as well as on land. This indicates that the powers were fully free, yet in orderly flow. They thus were establishing an interconnection between the unconscious and conscious. At this time I realized that healthy psychic development was underway.

It seemed to me that Christoph was a born electrician. He repaired the train, handled it with great skill and enriched it with all kinds of electrical details. In order to make it easier for him to stay home alone upstairs with his brother, I suggested that Christoph install a small Morse-code set which could operate from one floor to another. Sending signals back and forth created fun for both children and parents. While he was with me, I gave him the task of installing electric lights in my three-story dollhouse. Because a house is a symbol for man's inner being, I wanted him symbolically to light up his inner environment. Christoph was thrilled with his work. With great concentration he threaded the delicate wires and mounted the tiny lights and switches. After several hours work, all the lights in the six rooms could be turned on and off. The amazement over Edison's invention of the electric light bulb in the last century could hardly have been greater than the effect on Christoph when all the rooms of the dollhouse could be lit up at once. On top of that, it was his own work!

This gave rise to a further sand picture [Illustration 19]. A musician sat playing a harmonica on a small hill in the center. Circus figures moved clockwise and counter clockwise around the hill within a closed circle. Roman chariots, elephants, tigers, and horses, as well as clowns and an acrobat, were elements of the circus. The spectators were placed outside to the left and right. The Self, revealed in the preceding picture in the square form of the water area, the bridge and the movement of transportation in all four directions, had now clearly and significantly developed into a circumambulation around a center.

To clarify my strong emotion about this event I would like to go into the symbolism of the circumambulation. In Latin, "circus" means "ring" or "circle." In ancient Rome, the circus served principally for the Roman chariot races, and later for animal fights. During the Christian persecution, the Christians were sentenced to

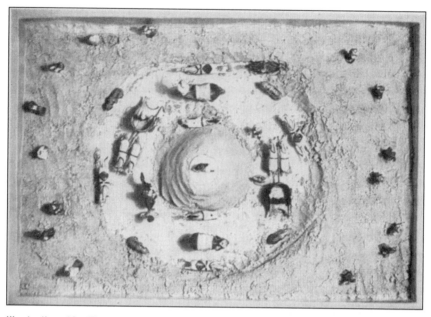

Illustration 19: The square from the last picture becomes a circumambulation around the center, as circus performers simultaneously move clockwise and counter clockwise. The Self is manifested, activating a powerful transformation.

fight the animals in the arena. Was it possible that this nine-year-old boy had heard of the Roman chariot races? Certainly not. Although he might have heard about it, living far from town in simple surroundings he never even had the opportunity to go to the circus. It was more likely that he had heard of trained animals like elephants and tigers, which circled around in the picture with the horses. Because it is not common to have Roman chariots in circuses today, we were confronted here with an archetype.

Christoph explained that the musician in the middle made music for everyone to enjoy. This picture is clearly concerned with a concentration toward the middle. On closer examination I saw that the two outer circles moved from right to left, or counterclockwise, which is psychologically comparable to a movement toward the unconscious. The inside figures inscribed a circle from left to right, or clockwise, which is the direction toward consciousness.

We know that a centering in man is a numinous experience.

That is to say, it is about coming into contact with his inherent religious forces. It is not farfetched to make an analogy between the circles in Christoph's picture and the three circular movements of the priest with the censer over the offering at a Catholic mass. The priest moves the censer twice from right to left and once from left to right, blessing the offering in preparation for the actual transformation. The boy's picture unquestionably represents a centering process, signifying a transformation. In Christoph's picture, in a seemingly unimportant game, the archetypal function of the healing psyche is expressed in a deeply moving way. Was it actually possible that the negative forces, represented in the picture by the Roman chariots and fighting animals, were about to be transformed through a still unconscious, but deeply religious, event?

The circle itself, and the circling around the central point in particular, has a godly character in other cultures as well. Jung mentions this in *Psychology and Religion*:

> Since olden times the circle with a centre has been a symbol for the Deity, illustrating the wholeness of God incarnate: the single point in the centre and the series of points constituting the circumference.
>
> Psychologically this arrangement is equivalent to a mandala and is thus a symbol of the self, the point of reference not only of the individual ego but of all those who are of like mind or who are bound together by fate. The self is not an ego but a supraordinate totality embracing the conscious and the unconscious. But since the latter has no assignable limits and in its deeper layers is of a collective nature, it cannot be distinguished from that of another individual. As a result, it continually creates that ubiquitous participation mystique which is the unity of many, the one man in all men.[11]

Christoph succeeded in creating a temenos in his innermost being by way of a transference that brought about a mother-child unity. In this way he was able to protect himself from any disintegration that might be feared from the representation in **[Illustration 17]**. From this protected space it was now possible for him to cope with the outer world. If we recall the first picture, the inside and outside were not in

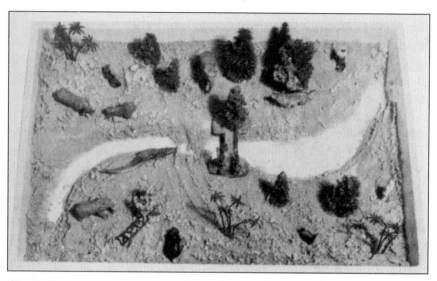

Illustration 20: Two dark-skinned figures stand to the right of a jungle that has a river running through it. The two men emerge from the shadows of the jungle as the ego begins to distinguish itself from the unconscious, instinctive level of awareness.

harmony. In the protection of his home he was fine. But up on the hill he felt terribly threatened. In his latest sand picture, he had symbolically expressed the centering that normally takes place in two or three-year-old children. From this point of centering, a strong and healthy ego should now develop.

Christoph became interested in painting and clay modeling, showing further skill with his hands and revealing a very good sense of color. During this phase, I gave him increasing opportunities to be active in a creative way. This is not a matter of creating perfect works of art, but of investigating ideas and trying to express them.

The developmental level of the infant that Neumann[12] mentions must be re-established during therapy. The first phase of ego development subsequently arises out of the security of the mother-child unity. This stage of development manifests itself as the vegetative, animalistic level. During this phase images of vegetation and of animals are often produced. It was like this with Christoph. His next picture portrayed a jungle **[Illustration 20]**. A river with natural banks flows through the middle of a wooded region connected by a ford and a bridge. Animals move toward the stream for a drink. On the extreme right on each side of the water stands a Moroccan. In these two dark-skinned people I saw the ego as it began to distinguish itself from the instinctive level dwelling deep in the unconscious, represented here by the jungle.

In daily life, Christoph was showing himself to be increasingly self-reliant. His ambition began to assert itself more and more. Good marks became important. I was invited to assist at an examination in order to see his progress for myself.

It wasn't long before this new tackling of his environment was expressed in a picture **[Illustration 21]**. Whereas the water in the former picture flowed between natural banks, this time it is channeled in a man-made canal. Ships move in both directions. On both sides, soldiers fight and dark-skinned men battle over the Suez Canal, Christoph told me. In place of the darker trees, which recall the jungle, there are palms that grow in the Near East and Southern Europe. Elephants are also present.

Let us imagine a jungle scene, such as we might find in Africa. If we look at it psychologically, we witness a scene on a deeper unconscious level than one that takes place in the Near East by a man-made canal. One can assume therefore that the ego development in the boy is emerging with more force. Moreover, the fight rages around a canal that was built by man, as a scientific project. All of this con-

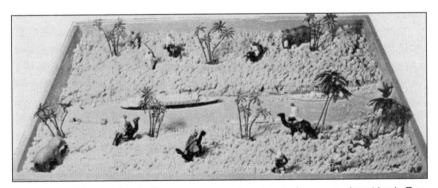

Illustration 21: Soldiers battle over a man-made waterway in a sunny desert land. Ego development progresses into the greater light of consciousness as Christoph experiences a growing readiness to become active and capable in the world.

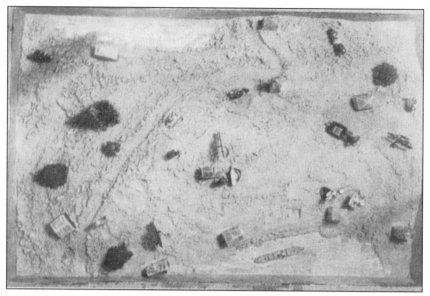

Illustration 22: Christoph now returns to his hill with freedom and security. He expectantly waits, "...for the bus to take me out into the world."

sidered, it seemed obviously important to encourage the boy in every way to do something that could be useful to him in a profession later on in life.

Among other things, on his own initiative he built a small funicular railway linking his friend's house to his own. However, he discussed all the plans with me and I offered him help in completing it. The funicular seemed to represent a link with the outer world that he needed very much for his future.

The school, which had caused so much worry in the beginning, was now hardly a prob-

lem. He worked with perseverance in the subjects that gave him the most trouble. The threat of being transferred to a special class had long passed. Even if he was not a brilliant pupil, he was certainly prepared for future professional or vocational training. The last picture **[Illustration 22]** that he made during therapy shows the hill that separates Lake Zurich from Lake Greifen. A few houses represent the villages, and the men near them are the inhabitants. A street winds around the hill. At the high point, at the top of the pass as it were, sits a boy. He sits in complete freedom on the hill, in the region where his

34

home is. This shows that the adjustment to the world is finally accomplished. The picture represents the transformation of the forces that were expressed by aggression in the initial picture. These were the influences that had hindered the child's development. Where fighting soldiers had formerly besieged the hill and had threatened the boy on his bench under the poplar tree, there now stood men who could pursue their work in peace. The boy, who saw himself in the first picture in a narrowly limited home situation surrounded by the din of war, was now waiting on the hill near the edge of the street for the bus that he said would take him out into the world.

NOTES

11. C. G. Jung, *Psychology and Religion: East and West*, Collected Works, Vol. 11. (New York: Pantheon Books, Inc., 1963), 276.

12. E. Neumann, *The Child*. (New York: G. P. Putnam's Sons, 1973).

CHAPTER 3

KIM:
Learning Problems
12-Year-Old Boy

Twelve-year-old Kim did not know how to enjoy his life. His father described him as lonely, withdrawn, without friends and often bored. Games had not interested him since his earliest childhood. Now and then he read a book but without any great interest. In the company of adults he appeared very well adjusted. His clothing was always correct and his hair neatly combed. Although he gave an impression of neatness, Kim worried his father. The boy's first school years passed without any great difficulties. Progressively, his withdrawal from comrades his own age became more obvious. Sometimes his learning abilities seem to be impaired. Kim was tested for intelligence and was found to have a good average. He started therapy but without notable success. The advice of the therapist was to send him to a boarding school, where it was hoped it would be easier for him to find friends of his own age with whom he could participate in sports and games. Kim's father did not want to be separated from his son. Since his wife's death several years earlier, he had clung tightly to Kim.

Here begins Kim's story. At the tender age of two, he lost his mother. A nurse undertook the task of raising Kim and his younger brother. For six years she played the role of mother to the boys and was loved by both. It was the father who appeared to suffer most from the loss of his wife. Time failed to heal his wounds, and his pain grew worse. He left the place where he had established his family and his work. Even more serious was the fact that he could not decide on a new field of work. A constant unrest had taken possession of him, and unrest means insecurity. In this condition how could he give the little boys the necessary security? Thus, on the advice of a therapist, the younger son was sent to a boarding school. Kim's father wanted to preserve what was left of the family relationship by remaining together with his older son. This was an absolutely understandable human wish that, in my judgment, should be accommodated, if it were at all possible.

According to his intelligence and ability, 12-year-old Kim was assigned to the first year of junior high school in a college preparatory program. He was not an outstanding pupil. Latin seemed to be most difficult for him. The question the troubled father raised with me was, "Will my son be capable of going through the junior high school without separating him from me?"

It is expecting too much from a therapist to answer a question like that with a "yes" or "no." Nothing is more complex, more delicate, and subject to countless influences than is the psyche. However, the development of the psyche's forces does emerge when a free, yet protected space is established. Only then will the psyche's possibilities become visible. When the psyche's possibilities do appear, we often view it as a miracle. The psyche has an inherent tendency to heal itself. The task of the therapist is to prepare the path for this propensity. It would be utter audacity to assert, on the basis of this inherent healing tendency, that the path will be found in every case. Nevertheless, as long as there seems to be the possibility for healing, every case is worth an earnest effort.

When Kim entered my therapy room for the first time, I got the impression of a boy who was not really young. I felt that what mattered in his life was bur-

The psyche has an inherent tendency to heal itself. The task of the therapist is to prepare the path for this propensity.

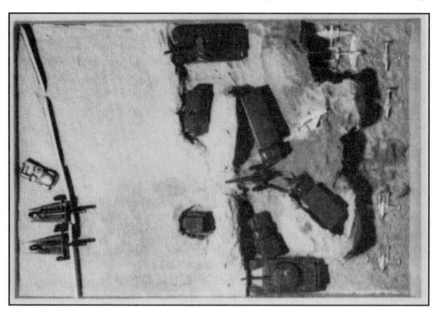

Illustration 23: The potential for transformation of a small trinity of forces confronts Kim's deeply entrenched fears and thwarted creativity.

ied deep within him.

Kim greeted me very politely yet somewhat inquisitively. Nothing seemed to disturb his correct attitude and behavior. I was convinced he would not play for the time being. I did not even dare to ask him to do so. This would make him even more unapproachable and probably would injure his dignity.

We talked of school and Latin, but after awhile, he began to yawn. That was the best possible expression for his complete lack of interest. For this reason, I knew that private tutoring would not help. Nor could a change of milieu bring about any substantial improvement of the situation. This listlessness was the expression of one-sided development, for which the cause still had to be found.

When Kim came to the second session, he acted much livelier. He asked me right away if he could build a barricade in my sandbox. Astonished by his own suggestion to play, I showed him the figures he could use. Something that had seemed to be impossible was about to be realized. First he carefully mixed the sand with water so that it could be easily formed **[Illustration 23]**. Then, with an unbelievable devotion, he built up walls that actually formed a whole system of barricades. With exact calculation, he put in heavy weapons such as tanks, cannons and bombers for defense, it appeared. At first, the left side of the sandbox remained empty. Only after he had again and again convinced himself that the weapons could not be seen from the other side was Kim content with the completion of the right side. Then he turned to the left side. Rather quickly he placed three light-artillery units behind a fairly weak tin shelter. He looked at the whole thing. Almost imperceptibly he added a final airplane that he defined as having crashed in the carefully built-up defense system.

The inequality of the opposed fields of force gave rise in me to the only question which I posed to the boy during the whole hour. "Can these three weak artillery units really withstand the heavy weapons?" His answer was, "One never knows." These

"Can these three weak artillery units really withstand the heavy weapons?"

His answer was, "One never knows."

words moved me deeply, for unconsciously he expressed the possibility of a healing in his answer.

The crashed airplane showed his situation. Until now his whole life was directed toward the conscious. He was intelligent. He could learn. He had acquired social manners and he was able to accommodate himself to everything imposed from outside. However, the creativity in him--that which really constitutes the essence of man--was nearly smothered. In the beginning phase of puberty, it is of extreme importance that access to the inherent energy sources that guarantee development of the personality be intact. In Kim's case this had been endangered since his early youth. Born out of the safe enclosure of the womb into the world, the child still requires the protection of the mother for a long time. Through the mother's care and, above all things, through the love she gives, the mother instills a feeling of security in the child. This is the only security that is necessary for the child to develop according to his own potential. If the mother is lost the child retreats inside himself. To protect himself against influences from the environment, he erects a bulwark around his innermost being. Fear hides behind this rampart. When it becomes too great it changes into aggression. If the aggression has no way to manifest and is repressed, it consumes so much inner energy that little remains for anything new in life. When this occurs, the child refuses to function when "too much" is expected of him.

For Kim, the demand that he begin the study of Latin was "too much." It is easy to understand how a sensitive child, frightened by a demand that seems too great, can lose courage and show a lack of interest in what is asked of him. This poses problems for parents and teachers alike.

The crashed airplane in the sand tray picture was an expression of the hopelessness Kim felt about his situation. The plane lay in that area where repressed aggression was represented in the form of heavy weapons behind the sheltering walls. This was the way Kim lived until the moment of his first sand tray picture. In fact, the sand picture--his first truly creative game-- began to animate his hardened demeanor. The three light-artillery units behind the insubstantial structure represent Kim's blocked dynamics. That there were three seemed meaningful to me, as three is a dynamic number. Wherever we meet the number three, it is associated with a course of events having a beginning and a goal. In fairy tales, for example,

The crashed airplane in the sandtray picture was an expression of the hopelessness Kim felt about his situation. The plane lay in that area where repressed aggression was represented in the form of heavy weapons behind the sheltering walls.

41

we know there are three difficult tasks that the young man must carry out in order to conquer his princess and finally win the kingdom.

Our boy had to reach his kingdom, too. For Kim this consisted of becoming a full individual in concert with his abilities and a useful member of the collective. Is not everyone his own master and king, enabled with talents and gifts to carry out tasks that revive him daily and make him happy? It does not matter what the field is. The king may work as a craftsman or in an intellectual discipline. What is important is that the king has his unique kingdom of gifts and abilities. Above all, it from here that he draws the almost more-than-human power he needs to lead and rule his kingdom.

In a further symbolic meaning, the number three holds a clue as to how this power is to be attained. Since ancient times, the number three is considered not only a dynamic force, but it is also defined as holy. Thousands of years before Christianity, acts of a divine nature were associated with the number three.

Thus, the number three seems connected with a super human power. In his psychological interpretation of *The Dogma of Trinity*, Jung says: "...the Trinity is an archetype whose dominating power not only fosters spiritual development but may, on occasion, actually enforce it." [13]

These divine energies were known to the unconscious of our boy. Under their protection the possibility arose for him to move beyond his evident weakness that was, in effect, bigger than the ego. Hope arose for a victory over his overwhelming aggressions. It is incumbent upon the therapist to intercept these powers as they manifest in a child. The therapist must protect them in order to foster the possibility of their becoming operational.

Again and again I am deeply moved by the discovery of how close the child's psyche is to spiritual and healing forces. The simple words of the child, "One never knows," were at the same time, an expression of a profound worldly wisdom. Kim's words reminded me of the Chinese sage, Lao-Tse. In Chapter 76 of Lao Tse's *Tao Teh Ching* we find a valid reminder for men in the West as well as the East:

Man, when he enters into life,

is tender and weak,

42

And when he dies,

then he is tough and strong.

That is why the tough and the strong are

companions of death,

the tender and the weak,

companions of life.

For this reason:

If the weapons are strong, we will not be victorious.

In Chapter 78:

That which is weak conquers that which is strong,

and what is tender conquers what is tough,

To everyone on the earth this is known,

but no one wants to act by this.[14]

Lao-Tse expresses the possibility that the weak may triumph over the strong. This has been proved in many examples throughout history where, through their deep faith, the weak have gained unsuspected powers that often led to their victory.

When Kim came to the next session, he wanted to build another bulwark **[Illustration 24]**. Delighted at his desire to play and excited by expectation of how his condition would develop, I gladly let him do as he pleased. A further barricade was made, but in a somewhat looser form. When he looked at it, he said, "This is not built up as much as before." As a

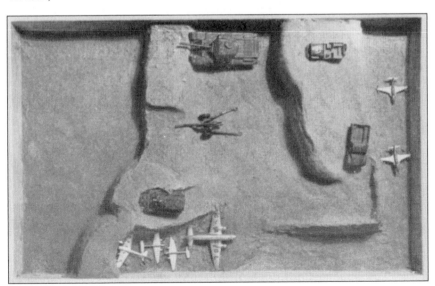

Illustration 24: Kim's defenses ease as the protective barricades begin to lessen.

matter of fact, the walls were no longer as high. It seemed as if Kim had already started to remove the protective walls.

In the following hour Kim went without delay to the sandbox [Illustration 25]. Walls were built again, but this time they formed a runway. Behind the walls airplanes and bombers were ready for take-off. The runway was big and wide. It was directed towards the left, the side of his yet unexperienced possibilities. This meant that the way was now open for his unusually intense aggressions. The blocks had been removed.

How would this happen in a boy who had never in all his life, consciously destroyed anything? I awaited the answer in excitement.

At the next sitting, Kim no longer wanted to play in the sand. When I asked him what he wanted to do, he looked around and discovered some darts. He threw them at the target meant for darts. However, after a short time it bored him to use the target and he began to throw the darts at my freshly painted paneled wall. Kim put so much energy into his throwing that the splinters fell

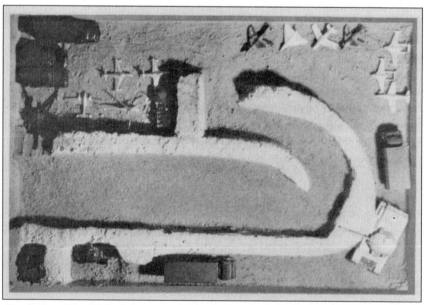

Illustration 25: Walls define a runway where Kim's intensely aggressive energies prepare for release.

44

from the wooden walls. Probably to his great amazement, I let him do as he liked. For the first time his features lit up. That I did not blame him nor express myself, to say for example, "It is terrible how you demolish my room!" gave Kim the assurance that there was something here which would help him.

The game with the darts was not enough, though. A small air gun seemed more attractive to him. Once again he began to shoot at a target and seemed to find pleasure in it, but he wanted to make noise, to hear clatter. At that moment, a thought came to me. We walked together through the wine cellar where many empty bottles lay. These could be shot into fragments. For a few hours this activity was his greatest delight. It came to an end, however, when there were no more bottles left. Now he had another wish. He wanted to shoot down the chandelier in the city theater. One

Instinctively, the boy had grabbed for a symbol of wholeness. By doing this he tended towards centering, so I let him do as he pleased. What I saw behind his destructiveness might not seem evident at first glance.

could readily recognize what enormous aggressions were still in the boy. That such a wish could not be fulfilled was also clear to him, yet he heartily wanted to break something that was still whole. As I felt that his aggressions were beginning to look for a goal, I gave him the freedom to choose an object in our room. The wildness that had found its expression in making simply noise, gradually faded into the background. He looked around until his eyes fell upon a little square wooden table in the doll house. He asked me if he could shoot at it. "Yes you may do that," I said.

At first it might seem that the little table from the doll house was a rather modest goal compared to the chandelier. The square of the table meant however, a wholeness.

Instinctively, the boy had grabbed for a symbol of wholeness. By doing this he tended towards centering, so I let him do as he pleased. What I saw behind his destructiveness might not seem evident at first glance. At this point, I would like once more to quote some thoughts from the Far East for further illustration. I thought of the spiritual meaning of archery in Japan. The art of archery is practiced there by many Zen masters. It is not about a bloody argument with a living opponent. It is a spiritual exercise, a dispute with oneself. When one aims at the center of the target, one aims at one's own center. In this way the archer tries to reach his own center. This is often a painstaking training that lasts for years. Herrigel says of this in *Zen und die Kunst des Bogenschiessens, Zen and the Art of Archery*,

> The competition comes into existence in that the archer aims at himself, and yet not at himself, and that he might hit himself, and yet not himself, and in this way, being the aimer and the target, at the same time, is also the aggressor and the victim. Bow and arrow themselves are only a subterfuge for what could also happen without them. It is the path to a goal, not the goal itself."[15]

Here we clearly experience what I mentioned beforehand. The quaternity, here the square table, appears when a centering as a sense of wholeness is sought. The boy was both an aggressor and a victim. He had to hit the qualities that hindered his development. In doing so, he hit himself. By taking this action, he replaced an old attitude with a new one.

A little figure belonging to the sand play was his next target. It represented a man who, in Jung's language, showed a true persona attitude. This figure had an attitude that is so perfect on the outside that it does not allow one to recognize what is going on within. He placed this little figure on a lump of clay and destroyed it completely with shots. In so doing he definitely overcame this same attitude that he had so far displayed himself. I must admit that I had to ask myself if I had not gone too far in letting this happen. I was almost afraid that he would now want to aim at living people.

The next day I asked Kim's father what effect these events had made upon the boy. "Something very out of the ordinary happened to me yesterday evening," he reported. "For the first time since earliest childhood, Kim gave me a goodnight kiss." Finally something had broken through the boy's rigid attitude. He had destroyed his mask himself. Emotions and feelings had broken through the blockade. As a result, he could embrace his father.

This moved me even more, because I knew that the father himself was incapable of spontaneously showing the child his own feelings. The father was overjoyed that it was now the boy who came to him.

Thus, the moment had arrived when the negative aggressions had been adequately lived out. It is not often easy to recognize this turning point, but it is one of the most important moments in therapy. If the therapist misses it, there is danger that energies

Thus, the moment had arrived when the negative aggressions had been adequately lived out. It is not often easy to recognize this turning point, but it is one of the most important moments in therapy.

which had been set free will become permanently destructive. For this reason it is extremely important that the newly awakened energies are caught by the therapist and led into constructive paths.

In the following hour, Kim discovered a blowtorch. At first he amused himself in the garden by letting the fuel in the torch drip to the ground, so that he might light it afterwards. He produced many little flames, and I admit it was a very amusing game. However, it was not what I was striving for in that moment. So I intervened to guide him for the first time in the therapy.

I explained to him that the blowtorch was a very useful instrument with which one could, for example, remove old paint from wood. My house was built in the Middle Ages. At the time there were still many beams that were painted an ugly color. Together we tried to remove the paint with the glowing jet of the blowtorch. Now this was interesting! The enthusiasm for this game, which had turned into work, lasted for hours. The same energies that dissolved the paint with the flame instantly took a positive effect as the beautiful old wood of the beams reappeared.

It seemed to me that the moment had come for a new sand picture, and Kim accepted the proposal with pleasure [Illustration 26]. With delight I saw that the tanks were no longer touched. For the first time colors, trees and people appeared in the picture. Where strong bulwarks had been erected, there now stretched a thin forest across the landscape. I did not trust my eyes! To the left of that, four Indian women with children in their arms sat around the fire.

The archetypal family situation had come to life. What had broken apart in earliest childhood had begun to unite again! What had developed negatively for years and had to disappear in the symbolic form of the destruction of the square table, had now

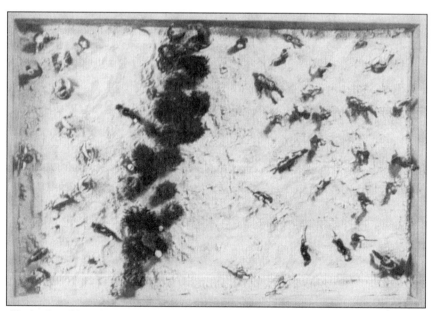

Illustration 26:   Kim experiences the positive qualities of the archetypal family as he touches the Self. The solidity of the four mothers provides the secure base he requires to heal in a positive way.

actually manifested itself in a wonderful way.

On the same side, four Indians in full-feather regalia stood in front of a totem pole, while a fight between cowboys and Indians took place on the other side of the little forest. "What do the Indians in front of the totem pole represent?" I asked. He answered, "They are praying that the fighting will end well for them."

There is no doubt that the symbolism in this picture is the appearance of what Jung calls the Self. The four mothers, as a symbolic representation of child-like wholeness in the most fortunate sense, show the transformation that happened with the boy. The limitless insecurity he was exposed to until then could now, on the basis of this solid and complete family, change into an inner security.

I was deeply touched by this happy change. From my experience, such transformation and revelation are always experienced as numinous. This was confirmed for me again in the form of the praying Indians. Life, especially in puberty, is perceived as a battle. However, if this battle is fought based on a deep-rooted security that contains a numinous quality, it develops and strengthens the total personality.

A week later Kim produced a similar picture **[Illustration 27]** that deepened the impression of the preceding one. Where four Indian women had formerly sat, now eight Indian figures with ceremonial pipes in their mouths surrounded the fire in a circle, while some of the Indian women cooked and some had their children in their arms. Here, the centering had been reached.

The number four represents totality and is connected in most cultures with the earth. It thus points toward a condition of reality. The circle, on the other hand, signifies heaven as a sym-

Life, especially in puberty, is perceived as a battle. However, if this battle is fought based on a deep-rooted security that contains a numinous quality, it develops and strengthens the total personality.

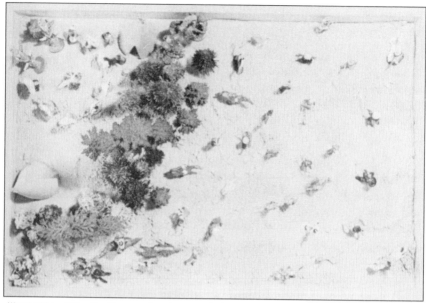

Illustration 27: Healthy ego development is initiated as Kim solidifies his spiritual center in the manifestation of the Self.

bol of totality and points toward the spiritual.

In my opinion, the manifestation of the Self, represented in many forms, but most impressively in the circle, means the starting point of healthy ego development. This is the beginning of the unfolding of inherent personality traits. Kim's healthy development now seemed safeguarded. The first manifestations of healthy development require protection and care, as with a newborn baby. Therefore it is wrong to dismiss a child from therapy at this moment. At this time the potentials for develop-

ment, which had formerly been inhibited by fears and experienced as aggressions, are set free. They must now be helped and directed. With the proper guidance and care, tasks that formerly seemed impossible and talents that could not express themselves can suddenly be approached with ease.

The many energies that were now awake in the boy were evident in a picture for which he used two sandboxes **[Illustration 28]**. This was a car race in which his favorite car was in the lead. With their strong motors, the racing cars personified his freed

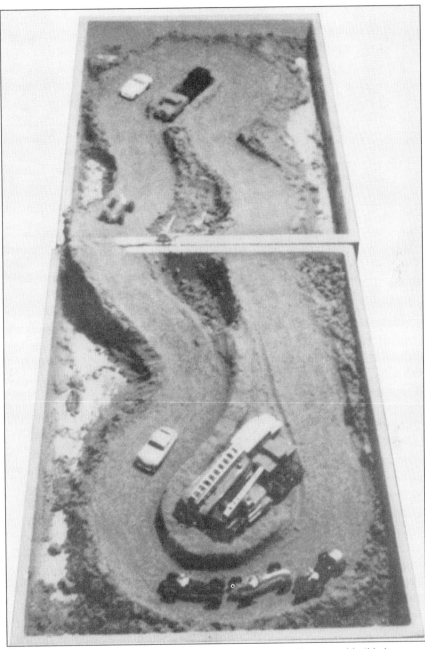

Illustration 28: Kim's capable adaptation to the outer world is secured in this large orderly race track.

powers. They moved safely in secure, orderly paths. Should they skid off the road, the fire brigade, the Red Cross and transport trucks stood ready. Where a crashed airplane lay in the first picture, indicating a disconsolate situation, there was now a helicopter standing ready for take-off. In reality, the boy had lived through three psychological stages. These were apparently indicated by the number three, the form of the light weapons on the left side. Symbolized here is the expression of the aggressions, the manifestation of the Self and a positive use of the energy sources. The goal, the king-dom that we wanted to reach, was at the point of being realized.

Kim found delight in constructive work. He made many friends and became a good friend to his father. At the same time, he started to assert himself at school. Today, six years later, and long since dismissed from therapy, Kim will shortly take his Matura exams to graduate from high school. Now, for himself, he can resolve the question that had been so difficult at the beginning of therapy.

NOTES

13. C.G. Jung, *Psychology and Religion: East and West*, Collected Works, Vol. 11, (New York: Pantheon Books, Inc., 1973), 193.

14. Lao-tse, *Tao-te-king, Das Buch von Sinn und Leben*, translated and annotated by Richard Wilhelm, Eugen Diederichs, (Dusseldorf/Koln, 1957).

15. E. Herrigel, *Zen in the Art of Archery*, (New York: Pantheon Books, Inc., 1953), 12.

SANDPLAY:
A Psychotherapeutic Approach to the Psyche

CHAPTER 4

DANIELA:
Passivity
12-Year-Old Girl

Daniela's mother described her 12-year-old daughter as shy and inhibited. She said that the girl lacked the courage to visit anywhere without her, and that Daniela was not even able to stay alone overnight with her grandmother. Mother said it was difficult for her daughter to make friends, and she was quite a lonely child. Her teacher complained of the child's lack of interest and participation in school activities. She reported that, in spite of the fact that Daniela was tall and physically strong, she gave the impression of being a completely powerless pupil. The teacher felt Daniela was unfit for the academic high school level to which she had been assigned, and the school proposed putting her through a less demanding course of study. Daniela's parents were very disturbed at this proposition, so they brought her to me for observation.

Daniela willingly agreed to my suggestion that she play with the figures in my collection. She started, as she said, by "...letting cows graze in a fenced pasture" [Illustration 29]. In front of the pasture she placed a coach pulled by two horses, whose hooves stuck deep in the sand. Directly in front of the horses she marked off a street leading to an inn on the opposite side. A man walks toward the inn. A bench for resting is placed by the street, under a tree.

It seemed apparent that Daniela's coach of life had come to a standstill. The horses could go forward only with great difficulty. The

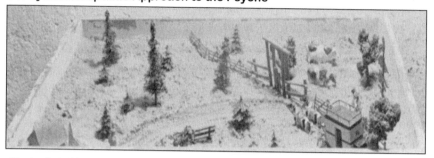

Illustration 29: Daniela's development is arrested by her mother's need to control, as she struggles to discover her own inner resources.

horses' hooves are mired near a motherly area represented by the grazing cows. The path to the outside world, here the inn--the place that is open to visitors-- appears long and tiring. The position of the inn in the far left corner directly opposite the pasture and the coach, indicates that the child needs to access her own unconscious, inner resources. It is essential that Daniela do this in order to be able to develop adequately. At the inn stands a male figure. Unlike the mother who embodies the world at home in the far right area, this male figure represents Daniela's relationship to the outer world.

Although Daniela gave the impression of being overly introverted, she seemed at ease with me from the start. To Daniela's parents, I suggested short-term therapy, in which I would try to liberate Daniela from her inhibitions.

In the second hour, Daniela reported that she had a "gruesome" dream involving snakes that she could not forget. I suggested that she draw or paint these snakes, since alarming things often lose some of their power to frighten when we attempt to reproduce them. She started the task immediately. With a sure hand she drew eight snakes dispersed in a meadow. She colorfully painted them with watercolors. The meadow was a luscious green, strewn with flowers. Daniela thought that the picture gave a rather gay impression. A slowworm rolled up in itself was the only snake tinted gray. This small harmless reptile might represent the problem still lying wholly in the unconscious. This colorless, gray serpent may symbolize an undeveloped, feminine aspect of the girl's being.

The snake often appears during puberty, when the transformation to adulthood penetrates into deeper layers of the psyche. The shedding of the snake's skin symbolizes a renewal in the unconscious that animates the secret of life.

I try to interpret dreams and sand pictures on the level of the child's conscious understanding. For this reason, I asked Daniela what number of subjects she had at school. Eight was the answer! Except mathematics, she said she managed all of them passably. We agreed that of the eight snakes, the single coiled serpent represented the most disliked subject, and that from now on, most of her attention had to be given to it. With that, the dream lost its menacing aspect for Daniela.

Daniela's second sand picture [Illustration 30] shows a traffic jam at an intersection. Cars approach from four sides, but the intersection is too narrow making it impossible for them to pass. Daniela explained that only the ambulance, which is right at the intersection, can pass through. It is striking that so many cars move down a tree-lined street from the left. It appears that that the un-

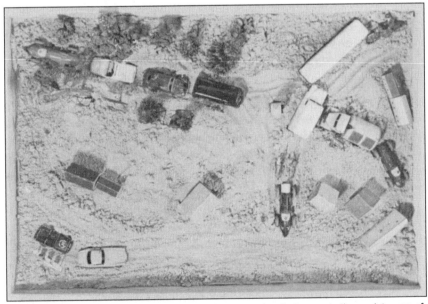

Illustration 30: Daniela taps new unconscious energies that come to the assistances of her blocked development.

conscious energies that were previously blocked are already in motion. This new flow of energy is supported by the gasoline station in the lower left corner. Here the motorists can refuel with new energy. The picture is a hopeful indication Daniela will be able to overcome her passivity. The ambulance that comes to the rescue in the intersection indicates that the quickening new energies can be properly directed and disciplined in therapy.

The third picture [Illustration 31] clearly indicates that the energies of life had started flowing. A wide stream crosses the landscape. A bridge over which cars can pass connects both shores. To the left is the inn. Now it can be reached by automobiles. Daniela brought some rather large stones from the garden and placed them in the river. The flowing water indicates that the restraints in her had started to dissolve. The stones signify the remaining obstacles that must be overcome.

This picture reminds me of a description of water in the Chinese *Book of Changes*, or *I Ching*. "Water sets the example for the right conduct under such circumstances (of danger). It flows on and on, and merely fills up all the places through which it flows; it does not shrink from any dangerous spot nor from any plunge, and nothing can make it lose its own essential nature. It remains true to itself under all conditions."[16]

The powerful, persevering nature of water conveys a strong sense of confidence regarding Daniela's future. Daniela needed this strength, as she was becoming much more active in her daily life. She met occasionally with friends and invited them to visit her at home. She found pleasure in doing handicrafts. Above all, she liked to paint and draw and showed real talent.

In her fourth picture [Illustration 32], Daniela depicts a circus. She divided the entire space into six squares. A performance takes place in each area. In the upper left, tigers and lions perform their tricks. The tiger leaves the podium while a lion is on the point of ascending it. In the adjoining area, the trainer occupies himself with four elephants. In the upper corner, five ballerinas form a circle. White horses circle around one who stands in the middle at the bottom left. A Roman chariot is in the next section. Clowns do their tricks on the bottom right of the sandbox.

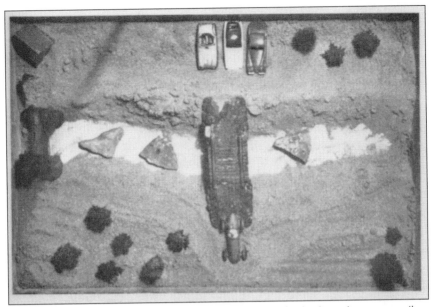

Illustration 31: Daniela's own powerful energies move freely along clear, open paths. She now has the power to develop in her own way and to handle the obstacles she encounters.

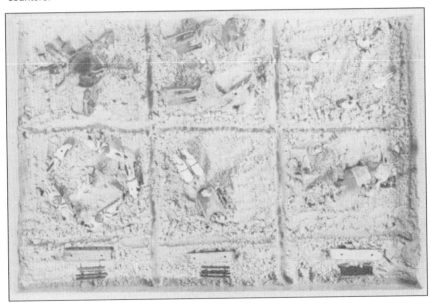

Illustration 32: An abundance of circles and squares reflect a deep centering in the Self as Daniela experiences her own true inner feminine nature.

Benches are arranged for the audience along the very bottom.

The different representations in the squares all represent a circumambulation or aim toward centering. Because it appears with the lion, the tiger can be seen as the feminine, shadow aspect of the lion. The Latin word *tigris*, the tiger, is of the female gender and stands for dark womanliness. The lion, as the king of the animals, is associated with the sun because of his yellow coat. The lion symbolically alludes to a clearing up of the conscious mind. The lion's vitality speaks for energies that are ready to awaken. Since the tiger descends from the podium in the center and the lion is on the point of ascending it, we can assume that this indicates a transformation in Daniela's development. This transformation will lead to a vitalizing of the energy forces that had until now, slumbered in the child. The elephants are also a symbol of strength and intelligence. Their presence in the adjoining square reflects Daniela's growing vitality.

The true femininity of the girl is expressed in the dance of the ballerinas. Walter F. Otto says in *Menschengestalt und Tanz, The Dance*, "Dances were originally the spontaneous expression of deeply stirred emotions where the cause and the result of the emotions become one."[17] The dancer merges into his own essence, into his divine essence. The circle of dancers in Daniela's picture indicates not only her femininity, but contact with the inner deity that lives in every human being. The circle has always been the expression for that very great experience that has been associated with the divine. Here in this picture, a 12-year-old girl presents a deep inner experience that could never be put into words.

Horses are animals with excellent instinct. Because they carry riders, they also have a maternal aspect. Symbolically, white horses are heavenly horses and are near the gods. The white horses encircling the one in the center that stands on its hind legs might thus express an unconscious religious tendency in Daniela.

Circular movement is reflected throughout this picture. The Roman chariot reminds us of the original meaning of the circus, as spectacle. The Greek word *kirkos* means circle.

The clown is a jester who possesses a thorough knowledge of artistic disciplines. Behind his jests hides profound, universal wisdom. The jester's riddles must be interpreted and made understandable by each individual. In this way the clown refers to the further development of Daniela's personality. This phase of personality development normally follows a period of inner peace and centering, which Daniela had abundantly expressed in her many circular movements around a central point.

Daniela's school work and general participation in school activities improved substantially between this session and the next. The picture she did a few weeks later **[Illustration 33]** showed that our prediction about her growth and development had been correct.

In this picture, five women come to the village well to fetch water. The well is underneath the large roof that appears just above the little forest. A man stands on the left. A path with a bridge over it leads to the nearby village. In contrast to the five circling ballerinas that assumed a numinous countenance in her previous picture **[Illustration 32]**, these five women carry out an

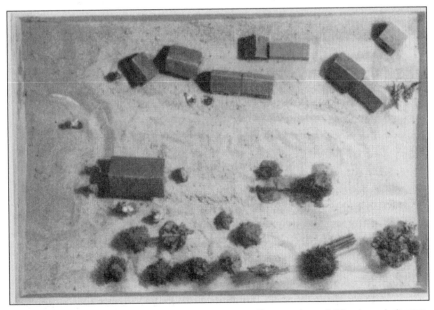

Illustration 33: Daniela's ego continues to strengthen as she solidifies her wholeness as a woman. The guiding influence of the animus is activated, and she has access to her own depths.

everyday chore. Natural womanliness is now present. This is the woman who can provide for the nutrition and welfare of her family. The image of the natural woman belongs to the stage of growth in which the transformation from girl to woman takes place. Daniela's ego is strengthened as she undergoes this phase of development.

Daniela has now reached the source of the unconscious that was foreseen in her first picture. In the image of the well, Daniela taps the source of her nature, previously concealed, but now brought to the surface. The action of drawing water from the well is like catching a fish. As a symbolic gesture, it brings contents from the depth of the unconscious to light.

The figure of the man standing somewhat to the side signifies the masculine aspect of

I repeatedly observe that the contra sexual aspect of the personality is activated directly after the centering experience. Only when the contra sexual aspect of personality is definitively activated can the individual form a proper relationship to the outer world, the collective.

the girl's being. He now assumes his important place in the formation of her personality.

I repeatedly observe that the contra sexual aspect of the personality is activated directly after the centering experience. Only when the contra sexual aspect of personality is definitively activated can the individual form a proper relationship to the outer world, the collective.

Daniela's school problems resolved, and her relationship to her mother eased. She dedicated herself to drawing and made posters indicating that she was turning more and more to the outer world.

In her final sand picture [Illustration 34], Daniela proved her readiness to leave the parental nest. On an airfield, planes stand ready to take off. Ships ride at anchor ready to sail away. A mail coach and a car stand ready to start and a train begins to move. Daniela was ready in all dimensions, the water, the land and the air, to explore the four points of the compass.

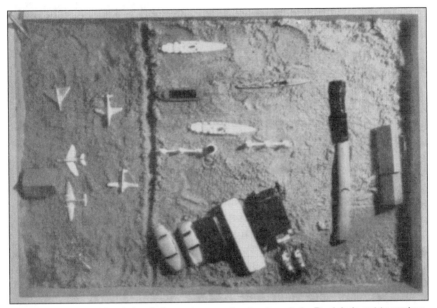

Illustration 34: Ready in all dimensions--water, land, and air--Daniela is set to explore the four points of the compass.

NOTES

16. *I Ching, Book of Changes*, R. Wilhelm & C.F. Baynes, Trans., (Princeton, NJ: Princeton University Press, 1971), 115, Hexagram 29.

17. W.F. Otto, *Menschengestalt und Tanz* (Munich: Hermann Rinn, 1956).

CHAPTER 5

CHRISTIAN:
Enuresis
12-Year-Old Boy

Generally it is very difficult to cure enuresis. It is especially difficult when the child is older and is expected to have outgrown bedwetting. You can imagine my great doubt when a mother phoned to ask if I could help her 12-year-old son with this problem during an eight-day vacation to my area. I finally gave in to her urgent request and agreed to see the boy in my office for consultation. I hoped to be able to get to the root of this complaint in our short time together. During his vacation, the boy stayed with relatives who lived close to me.

Christian was a very bright sixth-grade pupil. He appeared to be somewhat inhibited in the presence of his mother, who was the authority in the family. By contrast the father was rather indulgent. Christian relaxed immediately as we entered the playroom together.

Since I hoped to diagnose Christian's illness as fast as possible, and if at all feasible to give a prognosis, I immediately asked him to make a picture in the sand with my figures. This is not my usual procedure. Obviously pleased, he followed my suggestion, even though he appeared somewhat doubtful that this would help him be rid of his unpleasant habit. While he looked at the figures he started to talk. He told me that he suffered greatly from bed-wetting. Several doctors had been consulted, but no remedy was found. Christian said that he would always awaken after it was too late to go to the toilet. He said he had even tried a complicated mechanism to wake him up in time, but this had also failed. I felt sorry for Christian when he confided his difficulty to me. He evidently suffered very much. Again he shook his head. He did not understand how sandplay could help him. I explained that I might be able to discover the roots of his problem from his sand picture. I told him that this knowledge is based on long and thorough studies I have made, and that when I can discover the cause of his trouble, I might be able to help him. I further explained that we have much in us we know nothing about. Sometimes these are "good ideas" that can be helpful and sometimes these are "bad ideas" that cause disturbances. I ex-

plained to Christian that such images will come to the surface while he plays in the sand, and I hoped to be able to detect whether they had anything to do with the bed-wetting.

Wondering about this, he looked at me quizzically and began to choose some figures. He drew an oval in the sand with his hand and populated it with soldiers and crusaders [Illustration 35]. Christian stated that they are fighting with each other, and then he separated them with a high fence. They are being shot at from the outside by other soldiers, as well. A wounded man is carried away on a stretcher. Some Englishmen stand nearby apart

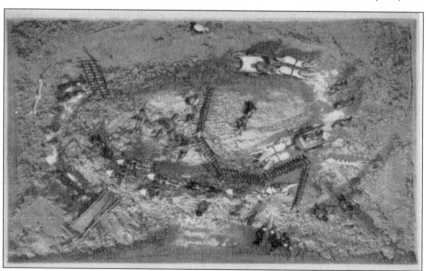

Illustration 35: Christian seeks inner stability to quell his critical inner conflict. A pelican holds the possibility for a secure mother-child unity.

from the battle. Christian said they will help bring peace. At the midway point near the upper rim of the sandbox, he placed a pelican.

From this picture, I could readily recognize the warring, oppositional energies inside Christian. They produce insecurity, and therefore he feels threatened from the outside. He even portrays himself as a wounded soldier, who is hurt and has to give up the fight. However, the situation is not completely hopeless. Christian said the Englishmen will achieve peace. He was unable to tell me why only the English would be able to bring peace. He simply remarked that he liked them very much.

For my interpretation of what this might mean, I resorted to the generally accepted characteristics of Englishmen. The character of the English people has been molded through the centuries by their insular location and the stability of their society. The English appear to be self-confident and balanced. The entire world is familiar with the English concepts of "the gentlemen" and "fair play." These qualities figure prominently in the emphasis on character development that plays an important role in English education. We can see from these associations that Christian longs for an inner stability. I wondered what the meaning of the pelican that oversees this entire event might be. A pelican is a symbol of motherly love. According to an ancient legend, it tears open its breast to nourish its young ones with its own blood. I wondered if this might indicate that Christian unconsciously expects the restoration of his inner peace to occur in the protection of a mother-child unity. I could see that Christian's first sand picture points toward a mother-related problem.

Christian's mother told me that she was solely responsible for the upbringing of her four boys. She said that she had to discipline them and teach them orderliness, because their father was completely consumed by his profession. She said he spoiled the children during the rare times they were together.

The following day, Christian made another sand picture [Illustration 36] that provided even more insight into the problem. It represents a circus. An animal trainer is in the arena with four tame tigers. Christian positions a lamp with four arms in the center. This is a very unusual item for a circus arena. Spectators are all around. On the left artists, clowns and Roman chariots are ready to perform. This picture made it clear to me that Christian experienced his mother's instruction as "taming." She had assumed the tasks of a father with a lot of strength and energy, but Christian yearned for warmth from his overly conscientious mother.

Recognizing what his situation was, I undertook to follow his lead entirely. He soon began to feel at home with me and wanted to play with other materials. Since it was close to Christ-mas, Christian wanted to use this opportunity to make some Christmas presents. He worked with clay and succeeded in making a very nice bowl. He became gay and alive as he painted it. I was so happy to see this liberation in Christian. Because he had unconsciously communicated his problems to me in his two sand pictures, this release was set in motion.

After working on his handicrafts two more mornings, Christian made another sand picture **[Illustration 37]**. This one was completely different. With great care, he built a firm, solid road

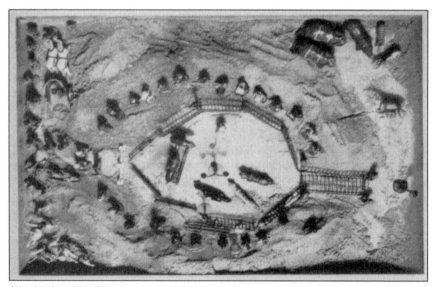

Illustration 36: The suppression of Christian's instinctual energies is clearly illuminated in the central arena for all to witness, as more spontaneous qualities prepare to emerge from the unconscious.

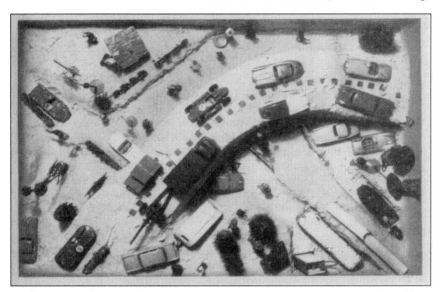

Illustration 37: Christian's energies now flow in an orderly fashion, as healing forces move into a prominent position.

with an underpass. This was rather difficult to do. It required an elaborate wood construction that would hold the sand he put on top of it. Soundly constructed, heavy traffic moves in both directions. The traffic flow is regulated by a strong, visible stripe down the middle of the broad road. The street that leads to the underpass is also bustling with vehicles. This traffic is directed by police. In this picture we see that the hostile energies portrayed in Christian's first picture are now well ordered and have lost their aggressiveness.

The pelican from the first picture is now replaced by a nurse, who has moved to the opposite side of the sandtray. I knew from this that Christian felt completely accepted by me. This simple acknowledgement initiated a profound healing influence on him. In the experience of being fully accepted Christian felt the security and protection of a caring mother.

The following day Christian played with craft materials. As he was busy building a small airplane for his brother, he suddenly said, "Mrs. Kalff, you know more than a doctor."

"How do you mean that?"

69

I asked.

"I have not wet my bed now for two nights," he answered.

I was very glad for him and quietly hoped that the bed-wetting would not recur. He no longer doubted that sandplay could be as helpful as the pills that he equated with the doctor. As there seemed to be some success in the treatment, I talked with Christian about the possibility of getting permission from his teacher to extend his stay. He loved this idea and we were able to extend his visit eight days. Christian came daily and continued to make Christmas presents for his brothers and parents. We never discussed his bed-wetting, but one day he shook his head repeating, "It is really true. You know more than doctors."

His bed remained dry. He spoke about his brothers and parents, and I felt his affection for them. He even felt secure enough to hope that he could go with his friends on a skiing trip after New Year's day. This would be a wonderful event, for until now he had had to stay at home because of his bed-wetting.

Christian was unable stay away from school more than two weeks. On our last day, I asked him to make another sand picture [Illustration 38]. Again it is a circus. However, this time the Englishmen are the featured actors in the arena. They now represent his own inner peace. I could scarcely believe it myself. A transformation had apparently taken place in this short time. I feared that the sudden interruption of our intimate relationship might produce a regression, but when he said goodbye, Christian whispered into my ear, "You really know more than a doctor."

For a while Christian phoned every week. Slowly, the intervals of our contact became longer and longer, until they finally stopped.

70

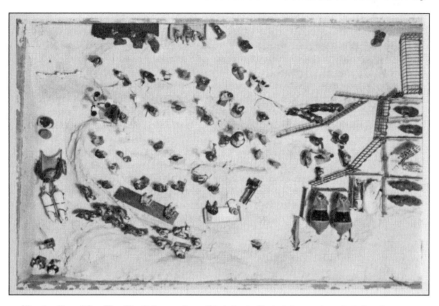

Illustration 38: The Englishmen from Christian's first picture return to bring the peace they promised. Now in the central arena, this deep sense of inner tranquility replaces his formerly powerless condition.

SANDPLAY:
A Psychotherapeutic Approach to the Psyche

CHAPTER 6

JAMES:
Early Trauma
16-Year-Old Boy

Sixteen-year-old James was exceptionally tall for his age. His shoulders were as broad as a man's, and his manners were more those of an adult than of a child. He smoked incessantly and carried on a lively conversation. His motto was, "Have as many friends as possible in order to never be alone."

James was the second oldest of five children. His entire family had come from the United States to live in Europe for a year. The children were to attend German-speaking schools to have closer contact with the people and culture of a different country. In America, James had problems with learning and concentration. In fact, he was barely able to manage his high school requirements. It was easy to foresee that he would fail in the rigorous curriculum of a foreign school. Above all, his English did not correspond with the norm for his age. It seemed highly unlikely that he could be accepted for admission to college. Due to their great concerns, James' parents asked me to let him live with me during the first part of their stay in Europe.

The great unrest that dominated James became apparent right away. He could not be alone, nor could he occupy himself with any activity. He thus led a very extroverted life. He went to a movie almost every day or met with friends in a cafe. To be "at home" was torment for him. However, it was immediately evident to me that his extroversion

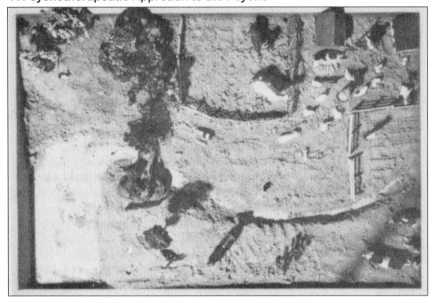

Illustration 39: James's instincts are locked away and unavailable as a result of early wounding in the mother-child relationship.

was not genuine. The gestures that accompanied his conversations revealed a helplessness and, in spite of his apparent nimbleness, his gait was heavy. His feet appeared to cling to the floor as though they sought to find a foothold on the ground. I wondered what might cause James to hide behind this adult façade.

At the beginning of our therapy, James produced a sand picture **[Illustration 39]** representing a rural scene. There is a farm with geese, chickens, and a sow with her young. A farmer sows his newly plowed field. Two horses, one light and one dark, are in an enclosure. There are blossoming trees and grazing cows. The terrain traverses a little stream that empties into a lake at the lower left. The whole picture gives a very peaceful impression. I wondered if it was an expression of the boy's longing to be close to nature.

At the same time two things struck me. Where the cows graze near the luscious green trees in the field, two ravens sit on a small leafless tree. In many early cultures such as Mesopotamia, Egypt, China, and still today in India, the mother cow symbolizes the nourishing mother. In this picture, the realm of the grazing cows could readily be seen as motherliness. As the leafless little tree is in the range of the grazing cows in James' picture, I was inclined to assume that something was disturbed in the mother-child relationship. Consequently, I asked James' mother if any experience or serious illness had taken place during the first year of his life that could have had an influence on his development. She remembered that when James was nine months old, he had bronchitis that was treated with inhalations. Through careless handling of the inhalator, the crib caught fire. Luckily, the baby was not seriously burned and had only a little scar on the forehead as a result. At this tender age the child still lives unconsciously within the mother-child unity. A trauma like this could have a disturbing effect on the relationship. I assumed that this experience produced a shock in James. I wondered if it were possible that the fire had so threatened James' early security

I wondered if it were possible that the fire had so threatened James's early security that he was unable to develop in a healthy way.

that he was unable to develop in a healthy way. I would need to find further clues to establish this conclusion.

The two horses in the picture are completely enclosed by a fence that has no opening or gate. The symbolism of the horse has many layers and can be viewed from different angles. The horse is a symbol of the instinctual sphere. Regarded this way, it is closely connected with man in the relationship between horse and rider. In fairy tales the horse leads the lost prince home. The horse is often considered clairaudient and clairvoyant. These capabilities make it a leader of lost souls, or psychopomp. A dark horse is associated with Poseidon, the Greek god of the sea. According to mythology Poseidon stirs the sea with his trident. Pegasus, the winged horse of Greek mythology, opens the spring Hippocrene with his hoof. For this reason, we attribute to him the ability to bring the unconscious water to light. Horses further symbolize psychic energies because of their fast gait and their intensity. We commonly call this "horsepower."

The white horse is symbolically associated with light and the sun. White horses pulled the chariot of Helios in Greek mythology. In the East it was a white horse that carried the monk with Buddha's scriptures to India. When the monk returned to China, a temple was dedicated to the horse. The white horse is found in the Christian tradition. In the Bible's Book of Revelations, 19:11, it says that Christ will ride on a white horse to fight the two evil animals that will come out of the nether world.

In James' picture, both the dark and the light horses are completely isolated from the rest of the farm. From this we can easily see that it is a loss of instinct that is chiefly to blame for his one-sided development.

In James' picture, both the dark and the light horses are completely isolated from the rest of the farm. From this we can easily see that it is a loss of instinct that is chiefly to blame for his one-sided development. He was unable to attend school in this condition. It was important that he become ac-quainted with the German language, so a student began tutoring him. It seemed to me that the most important thing was to try to provide him access to his instincts. Since he loved animals, I inquired about a position for him as a volunteer at the zoo. We were lucky when we discovered there was a job available. James had just passed the prescribed age of sixteen and carried the necessary insurance.

He went to the zoo two or three afternoons a week to clean the monkey cages. After doing this work, he watched the animals. This task was evidently fun for him. Little by little the animals recognized him and challenged him to play with them. One was very fond of James and reacted affectionately to him.

I looked through James' schoolbooks as a way of orienting myself to his level of school functioning. The torn books gave the impression of belonging to a boy who was bored. He had scribbled all over the margins. In the last blank page I discovered a small drawing by James that repre- sented Christ on the cross. However, this male figure had no penis. James could not have repre- sented his situation more clearly. Since his masculinity had not been able to de- velop, James saw himself as crucified. James appeared to be very attached to his mother. He was her favorite son. In fact, he was so en- tirely devoted to her that his own being had not been able to develop.

A dream that James related to me confirmed my apprehensions. He dreamed that the path which led to his house was lined to the left by crocodiles. Crocodiles have a threatening, aggressive, even devouring aspect. Since the crocodile lives in the water and on

the land, it represents a connec- tion between the unconscious and consciousness. In *Symbols of Transformation,* Jung mentions that such theriomorphic symbols always apply to unconscious libido manifesta- tions. Jung notes that symbols that appear as beasts either belong to the unconscious in gen- eral or point to sup- pression of the in- stincts. Referring to the instincts, Jung says, "... (they) are the vital foundations, the laws governing all life. The regres- sion caused by re- pressing the in- stincts always leads back to the psychic past, and conse- quently to the phase of childhood where the decisive factors appear to be, and sometimes actually are, the parents".[18]

James was in danger of being attacked and devoured by the crocodiles. To be able to deal with them, it was essential that he con- tact his own instinctual nature. I

"The regression caused by repressing the instincts always leads back to the psychic past, and consequently to the phase of childhood where the decisive factors appear to be, and sometimes actually are, the parents."

C.G. Jung

hoped that his relationship with the animals at the zoo, especially with the apes that had become his friends, would result in an awakening of those energies that still slumbered deep in his unconscious. Only when he became familiar with this energy would he be able to put it at his disposal.

Now that he was separated for the first time from the emphatically extroverted mother who controlled all his actions, it was frightfully difficult for James to orient himself. Even so, he quickly became happy in our house and tried to adapt himself to our habits. I attached great importance to reliance upon his own views in order to cultivate a feeling of his real self. The tutoring that he had been receiving almost daily helped him so much that soon he could converse a little in German. He could not and did not want to write, not even in English, for it required extraordinary effort, and his writing was practically illegible. Only unwillingly did he bend to my proposal of writing down a dream or an experience. A little later he visibly calmed down and began to show more interest in his own language.

Two months later, James came home and announced, "I told the zoo director that I was not going to work at the zoo any longer." I was somewhat astounded by the decision he had made on his own, yet I respected it. When I asked him what he wanted to do, he answered, "I want to go to school." This was even more surprising. We immediately discussed the question of which school, since he still had to accustom himself to the German language. Within a few days he began attending a private school as an auditor. Meanwhile, he continued his German classes with increased effort. During this time he produced a sand picture **[Illustration 40]** that indicated the unexpected change in his condition.

In the lower left corner is a small village. A rather wide path leads out of the village across the picture toward the top. A girl drives some geese home, and a shepherd is about to take the young lambs out of the fold and bring them to the pen. Grazing sheep, a horse and a cow walk toward the village. It is evening. A small group moves on the path toward the village. A man and woman walk with a donkey. I asked James if these people had any meaning. He said they were Mary and Joseph on their way to the village, because Mary was

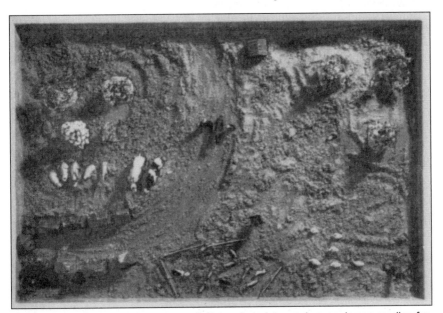

Illustration 40: Preparations are made for a deep introversion, as James readies for rebirth in the protective care of the archetypal mother.

about to give birth to a child.

This statement moved me deeply! I wondered if it could be possible that James, who until now had apparently been thinking only of getting away from himself, was already on the path to finding himself. I wondered if the child that was to be born could be the arrival of new conditions in himself. I wondered if it was James himself going to be newly born. I saw some signs in the way he spoke of his friends or the animals in the zoo. I saw the healthy way he had established his relationship to me. These observations along with James' picture left no doubt in my mind that he was about to approach a centering in the unconscious in much the way it takes place in a small child.

Even though the birth of Christ represents a one-time historic happening, it has an archetypal character. Jung says,

As the Logos, Son of the Father, *Rex gloriae, Judex mundi,* Redeemer and Saviour, Christ is himself God, an all-embracing totality, which, like the definition of Godhead, is expressed iconographically by the circle or mandala.

...As a shepherd he is the leader and the centre of the flock. ...In his human manifestation he is the hero and God-man, born without sin, more complete and more perfect than the natural man, who is to him what a child is to an adult, or an animal (sheep) to a human being.[19]

In this picture, young James expresses the approach to his own inner religiosity. According to his tradition it carries a Christian character, even though religion had not been consciously nurtured in the family.

James is on his way to surrender his care to the hands of the archetypal figure of the mother. In the picture it is Mary, the mother of God that is on her way to the birth. The shepherd is also about to bring the young sheep into safety before night falls. The evening calm and the preparations for the night when the great event is about to take place are signs of a significant introversion. This is a time of readiness for James to venture to the deeper regions of the unconscious.

In an effort to improve his English skills, James was given an assignment to write either a diary or a story of his choice every day. Over a period of time he wrote the story of a young man named *Tol* who, armed only with a knife, left his family to go into the woods. I want to quote the principal part of James' story here, word for word:

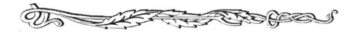

The Journey of Tol

Tol stopped a moment to watch the sun slowly creep over the treetops. Half smiling, he picked up his knife and trotted on down the hill. Upon reaching the bottom he branched off to the left, preferring the shelter of the trees to that of the open plain. He walked quickly, hoping to reach a small stream soon, for he was thirsty. After going a half mile he suddenly stopped. Changing directions, he moved slowly on. He had gone only a few yards when he stopped again. Frowning slightly, he moved on a little faster. After going several yards, he halted abruptly. This time there was no mistaking it! The sound of men! Soon the air became stagnant with their smell. He quickly sprang to the safety of a low hanging branch and then climbed up higher. The men soon came into view, shuffling along in single file. They marched past Tol's tree, then went out of

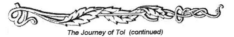

The Journey of Tol (continued)

sight. As soon as they were gone, Tol jumped down from the tree and darted off in the opposite direction. He ran until he had shaken off the sound and smell of them. Slowing down, he changed directions until he was parallel to the direction in which the men were going. He then kept up a steady trot until midmorning, when he came upon a small stream. Stopping only long enough to get a drink, he moved on.

He traveled the rest of the morning in peace, stopping only once to get a drink of water. By noon he was feeling very hungry, so he veered to the left and stepped out into a large plain. He stood in the tall grass for a while, getting used to the bright light and at the same time looking for food. After a time, he spotted a small gazelle a little away from the main herd. The wind was favorable and he was able to get within a knife's throw of it. In almost the same movement he threw the knife and chased after his prize. It was still kicking when he got to it, but he swiftly broke its neck. Carefully he cut off a piece and began to eat it. After eating all he needed to fulfill his hunger, he lay down on the grass to sleep, but before falling asleep his thoughts were, as always, of home.

Twenty days later:

Falling asleep, Tol began to dream. He walked up to the path to the cave and saw his wife sitting at the entrance, playing with their seven-year-old son, Ruk. Upon reaching the top of the hill, he looked around. The trees were just beginning to turn green, and the sweet fragrance of new flowers was in the air. Down in the valley he could see the movement of large animals as they plowed through the thick undergrowth. Here was the best hunting ground to be found within fifty miles. There were gazelles, bears, great mammoth and birds of all kinds. Fruit and water were near. His chest swelled with pride as he beheld all of this. This was his home, his will to live, and his very life. All that he could want or need was here. He turned around and called out to his wife and son, who were still unaware of his presence. Ruk, getting to him first, wrapped his small arms around his father's neck while his wife, a little slower, greeted him with tears in her eyes.

Still in the process of waking up, Tol could hear the joy of his wife and child over his return. Very reluctantly, he got up and started on his way again.

Fourteen days later:

Tol traveled the rest of the afternoon in comparative peace. As darkness of night came over the earth, he began to hunt for a tree in which to sleep. After a long and hard search he found an old, strong tree to climb up for shelter. He went up as far as he could then lay across a thick branch. As he lay there waiting for sleep to come, he tried to distinguish the different sounds of night: the loud and shrill cry of a pterodactyl flying around looking for food; the grunts of a tyrannosaur sleeping nearby; the voices and grunts of the smaller ani-

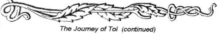
mals as they ran through the night in their endless quest for food.

He thought back over the days and weeks he had spent in search of Kezz, the horse. He had first seen him two weeks ago near the cave and had been trailing him ever since. But the trail had been lost when he had gone beyond the mountains. He had then been forced to turn toward home, where his wife and child patiently waited for him.

Soon his thoughts were only a confused jumble of ideas, and then he went to sleep.

Seven days later:

Waking early, Tol climbed out of his tree and stood in the sunlight listening to the birds high up in the treetops. How much difference there was between the sounds of night and those of the early morning! The morning was filled with the optimism of a new day, while the night was full of the sounds of struggle and laboring. The morning so intoxicated him that he had the urge to cry out to the world. Instead, he ran wildly through the bush without knowing where he was going. Quite suddenly he came upon a small lake and jumped right in. He enjoyed the cool water for awhile, then he sat down on the shore to dry off. A short while later, he saw a large head followed by a snake-like neck, emerge from the water. The creature took a deep breath then, with a loud hiss, sank back into the water. Having recovered, Tol began looking for food. Slowly he crept to the water. He stood

bent over the water for quite some time until he saw the fish he wanted. With unbelievable speed he dived after it, but the fish was faster still and vanished. He tried three more times, but without success.

On the fourth try, he was able to grab a fair-sized one, which he promptly knocked against a tree. Afterwards he rubbed it on a rock to scrape off the scales. Then he pulled the meat off the bones and, without great hurry, ate it in three bites. He then washed his mouth, picked up his knife and started off. The morning was marvelous! He felt like a dwarf as he ran between the trunks of the trees. Their tops were swathed in fog while the lower branches were covered by thick, green moss. He had the distinct feeling of being in a land of giants.

While Tol ran through the forest, other creatures were moving around him. A large brontosaurus was chewing grass. Nearby a small deer broke through the bushes. It was being pursued by a wolfish-looking animal. A pterodactyl flew overhead, looking for smaller animals. A wild tiger stood on a high rock and screamed its defiance to the world. Far off he heard the last cry of a small animal caught in the paw of a larger one.

None of this did Tol notice consciously, but rather all of it penetrated into his unconscious. When he heard the sound of a larger animal, he changed directions according to wherever the noise originated. This did not however, always work. Once he blundered through

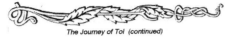

The Journey of Tol (continued)

the bushes upon a tyrannosaur and was lucky not to be torn between its jaws.

As he went along, his thoughts were turning over in an effort to figure out a way to capture the horse. He knew that when he saw him again he would have only one chance. For if he failed and hurt the horse in any way, there could be no hope of ever capturing him. Abruptly his train of thought stopped. He was not sure what was interfering, but there was something wrong. He stopped short. There in front of him was his horse, gleaming white in the morning sun. He was just twenty feet away, but Tol was sure that it had not sensed his presence. Very slowly the horse approached. When the animal was within ten feet, Tol quickly tried to devise a way to capture him. What he wanted to do most was to put him in some sort of enclosure, but he did not have the time to make one.

For awhile he was completely undecided as to what to do. Then thinking over the last days of his journey, he remembered a small valley that might be used as an enclosure. The big problem now was how to get the horse to it. By getting behind him and letting him smell his scent, Tol might be able to frighten him just enough to push him in the right direction. However, Tol did not want to scare the horse, for he might flee to the mountains.

Ever so slowly, Tol crept around behind the horse, taking great care not to step on any branches. At last he was able to get directly behind him. Cau-

tiously, he moved toward the horse. At first the horse took no notice, but when he got nearer the horse stopped grazing. As Tol came up closer, the horse moved away. This went on for about three hours until Tol was able to see the opening of the canyon, but he was afraid that the horse would not enter. But as Tol approached the animal, it gave no sign of being afraid of the trap to which he was led. Quite suddenly the horse moved on the rocky path that led into the canyon. As soon as the horse was inside, Tol began throwing branches across the entrance. The horse was his!

Now that he had the horse, Tol had to find a way in which to tame him. Tol knew that after he had trapped the horse, the animal would not trust him because he had been robbed of his freedom. To tame him he must first show the horse that he wanted to be his friend. Therefore, every morning he would bring small treats to the horse in the hope that he would be able to build up trust between them. At first, Kezz would become frightened and run to the far end of the canyon. But gradually Tol was able to stroke him while the horse nibbled small tidbits from his hand. After several days when Tol whistled, Kezz would gallop to him.

Many days went by before Tol decided that it was time to try the next step, which was to enter the corral with the horse. Very early in the morning Tol crawled under the gate and stood next to the horse. Kezz stood a moment, looking at his new friend, then trotted to the other

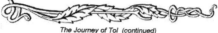

The Journey of Tol (continued)

end of the corral. Slowly, Tol walked toward him holding a large fruit in his hand and talked very softly. The horse stood for a moment, undecided as to whether to run away or stay. Finally, he decided to stay and he allowed Tol to stroke his neck. Every day after that Tol would enter the corral with Kezz, but never tried to get onto his back for fear of losing the trust he had built up so cautiously.

Several weeks passed, and Tol knew that sooner or later he must try to mount Kezz. He chose a fine spring morning and went to the corral earlier than usual. As soon as he was close to Kezz, the horse knew that something unusual was about to happen. Tol started talking to him and at the same time, tried to get up on the horse's back. Slowly, Tol mounted the horse. During all this time Kezz had stood perfectly still, but as soon as he felt Tol's weight on his back, he reared up and threw off Tol, who landed on the ground with a hard thump. Slowly, Tol got up and walked over to the horse, which had run to the far end of the corral. Again he talked softly to the horse, again he eased upon its back, and once more he was thrown off. Undaunted, he tried again and again, and with each try the horse would buck less and less, until finally Tol was able to trot around the corral without being thrown off. The horse was tamed! Tol jumped off, opened the gate of the corral and let Kezz out. He whistled, and Kezz came back.

This was the beginning of a long and true friendship between horse and man, which was to last for centuries.

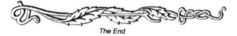

The End

In the story of Tol, James describes his own way of discovering his inner self. He left the outside world and had gone to the steppe and the primeval forest, that is to say, to the deepest layers of his unconscious. He describes very well how he avoided people. He wanted to be, and he had to be, alone with himself. Without knowing which energies slumbered within him, James had been oriented exclusively to the outside for too long a time. Step by step he describes the approach to the sphere of his animal instinct, symbolized by the animals of the steppe and the primeval forest. At first, he avoided them. Driven by hunger, he later had to learn how to deal with them. He hunted a wild animal, a gazelle, and ate enough of it to appease his hunger. In myth the gazelle stands for a picture of the soul. It is a shy, fugitive animal that is constantly in flight from the beast of prey. This part of his story clearly showed me how much James was threatened by overwhelming, aggressive instinct.

By eating until his hunger was quieted, he integrates much of his threatened, primitive self. In this way he is able to be on his guard and not fall between the teeth of a beast of prey.

Strengthened by a deep sleep in the branches of a tree, the following day he comes to a small lake where he had to exert great effort to catch a fish. To protect himself from the unfavorable devouring influences of his earlier surroundings, he had to fish his own hidden contents out of the unconscious water. The impending birth of Christ represented in his sand picture had already indicated that James was to be reborn. In *Symbols of Transformation* Jung says, "The fish in dreams occasionally signifies the unborn child, because the child before its birth lives in the water like a fish..."[20]

The fish caught and eaten by Tol is of great significance in James' development, for the story tells us that it is taken from the depths of the unconscious. James is thus enriched with the unconscious contents that the fish embodies. The fish is also a fertility symbol because of its many eggs. I wondered if James could be hiding an unknown treasure within.

Moreover, the fish is a symbol of Christ. Christ was often called by the Greek word for fish. Jung says that the fish symbol represents the bridge between the historic figure of Christ and the spiritual nature of man, in which the archetype of the savior reposes.

Unconsciously, James sought a deliverance from his condition. Now the means began to emerge from the depths of his unconscious. In fact, it looked as if the Self was beginning to appear as it does in early childhood.

After he catches the fish and ritually eats it, he discovers the tall trees that made a person feel very small. This part reminded me of a statement of the old Zen master, Suzuki. He said: "Western man wants to overcome Nature while Eastern man feels like a tiny part of her."

Only now was James really close to the earth. Animals

crept through the thicket, and in his joy over the magnificent morning in nature, he suddenly remembers the horse that he planned to capture. It was not long before he discovers it, *"There in front of him was his horse, gleaming white in the morning sun..."*

The security that James gained in his own instincts made it possible for him, with great caution, to catch the horse and to summon enough patience to tame it. I was deeply touched by his words, *"This was the beginning of a long and true friendship between horse and man."* With these words James is reborn and gains access to his instinctual sphere.

James understood that the completely one-sided attitude of his unconscious had led him astray. He knew that it was only according to the pattern of his own instincts that he could authentically develop his individuality.

At this time he told me the following dream:

"I was somehow together with my parents in search of Easter eggs. The peculiar thing was that we didn't find eggs, but presents. Contrary to my usual habit, I was nice to my sister. She received a horse and wagon that she wanted to drive around. However, I asked her if I could guide the horse. She agreed, and thus I drove my sister around in the wagon."

One of the most important Easter traditions is the gift of eggs, which are symbols of fertility. With this dream there was no doubt that James was advancing toward a more fruitful period in his development. The parents are present in the dream, but they do not participate in the activity. James himself now drives the horse that pulls his sister's wagon. The mother anima has lost power, as the sister--a younger anima image--gains new significance. The sister now becomes the source of new life. In *Psychology and Alchemy*, Jung comments about this transition. "This is really a normal life-process, but it usually takes place quite unconsciously. The anima is an archetype that is always present. ...The mother is the first carrier of the anima-image, which gives her a fascinating quality in the eyes of the son. It is then transferred, via the sister and similar figures, to the beloved."[21]

This remarkable transition was clearly evident in his everyday life. James expressed his wish to attend school as a student, in lieu of merely auditing classes. To validate the importance of these changes and to mark a new beginning, he once again switched schools. James registered for all the subjects that would enable him to pass the college entrance examination within a reasonable amount of time. Although German was still a handicap, he applied himself diligently to his studies and worked a great deal on his homework.

Soon James found a girlfriend, even though he was now almost always at home. James went out only once a week now, but his life was much richer.

One day James asked me spontaneously, "Mrs. Kalff, do you believe in God?" I told him that I not only believed, but that I had also experienced His existence. This was the beginning of many conversations of a religious and philosophic nature.

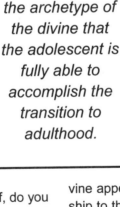

When the adolescent gains access to the realm of his natural instincts, the archetype of the divine appears. It is only in relationship to the archetype of the divine that the adolescent is fully able to accomplish the transition to adulthood.

When we work seriously with youngsters during puberty, we experience that a spiritual deepening accompanies their physical development. In former times among primitive peoples, the passage from one stage of life to another was consecrated through extensive ceremony. This was particularly the case in the transition from childhood to adulthood. Today these rituals have either lost their meaning or they have disappeared. For this reason, it is of great importance to deal with the question of God in therapy with juveniles. When the adolescent gains access to the realm of his natural instincts, the archetype of the divine appears. It is only in relationship to the archetype of the divine that the adolescent is fully able to accomplish the transition to adulthood.

A picture that James made in the sand about three

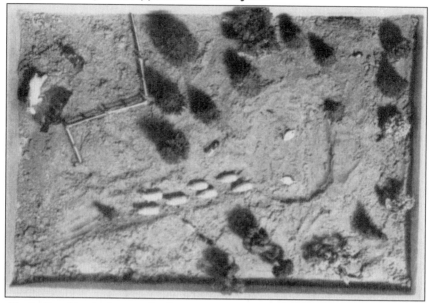

Illustration 41: As James gains free access to his instincts he forms a connection to the archetype of the divine.

months later **[Illustration 41]** confirmed my insights. It is a landscape. To the left stands a corral with two horses, a dark one and a light one. They are about to go toward the open gate. A shepherd is there with his herd. To the far right two swans swim in a pond.

The horses and the shepherd with his flock move to the left, in the direction of the unconscious. The introversion James had undergone when he wrote his story now exerts its effect. The horses are no longer locked in, as they were in the first picture. They are about to leave their corral and enter into relationship with the

world. This means that James is close to his instincts and has access to the outside world in accordance with his authentically introverted nature.

The herdsman is likely a symbol of Christ, as the good shepherd with the sheep.

In James' first picture, two ravens sat on a barren tree. Viewing them from their negative side we could have easily regarded them as birds of ill omen. It is true that James was an unlucky fellow. He had simply disguised his melancholy regarding his powerlessness with an emphatically extroverted demeanor. On their positive side, ravens are also friends of the hermits. They are messengers of the gods that bring help to people living in seclusion. In the Bible ravens are referred to as a bird of God. God responds to the calls of the young ravens in need. (Psalms 147:9; Job 38:41)

The raven symbolizes a bearer of light for some Indian tribes in James' native country. In James' initial picture, the ravens unconsciously indicate the road to be taken in therapy. The light shines brightest where darkness is deepest. James had to leave his overly rational sphere of consciousness in order to find the light that would illuminate his creativity in the inner self.

The swans that appear in [Illustration 41] announce this brighter possibility. In *Symbols of Transformation,* Jung mentions that "swan" derives from the root *sven,* the same as "sun" and "sound." He says that the swan signifies re-birth and new life.

The light shines brightest where darkness is deepest. James had to leave his overly rational sphere of consciousness in order to find the light that would illuminate his creativity in the inner self.

When it embodies as a sunbird, it is bright and clear and indicates an expansion of consciousness. Seen this way, the swan has to do with realizing inner possibilities.[22] By the same token it embodies a completely different feature. As the sunbird, a bringer of light, the swan has a premonition of what is in the future. It can see ahead to what is beyond the light and yet in the darkness. When we have a bad feeling, we frequently say: "I have dark forebodings." At this point in James' work, we cannot tell which of the two aspects of the swan will prove more significant.

James continued to work cheerfully toward his examination. One day he enrolled for the test, not to try to pass, but, as he expressed it, "to see how much is required." After some time, word came that he actually had passed the examination! Our joy was great, for now a college career was open to him.

Along with this success

89

another question emerged. How would he feel in his native country when, after more than two years abroad, he had grown accustomed to our way of life? He considered going by freighter, which would take several weeks. In this way James thought he would have time to prepare himself for the future and what might be different for him there. His parents, who wanted to celebrate what their son had accomplished, decided differently. They sent him a plane ticket and wanted him to get home as fast as possible!

It is not surprising that the thought of such a quick transition from one world to the next brought about something of an inner panic in James. He dreamed,

"I was in my native city, in a big house. A fire seemed to have broken out. God was there, but for some reason He could not help. Then the "man in the moon" was called. I saw him as he came from far away out of space. He and God went into a room and held council. What followed was unclear."

The fire that had broken out indicates the state of James' inner emotion. God by Himself could not help. Yet who was this "man in the moon" who was sup-

posed to assist God? There are endless variations in legends and myths about the "face" in the moon. Many tell of people carried off to the moon as punishment. I recalled a northern German legend of a big man who bends to pour water on the earth to extinguish a fire at ebb tide. This myth felt meaningful to me in the context of James' dream and his early experience of the fire. The moon has its effects on the ebb and flow of nature in the myths of almost all peoples. In contrast to the hot glowing sun of daylight, the moon embodies the water principle.

In a Chinese fairy tale, the man in the moon is described as sitting on a blooming, scented cassia tree. In Africa, the sweet pulp of the cassia is called manna. Manna was the food sent from the heavens to the Israelites in the desert. Manna is said to have fallen from heaven at night, at the same time as the dew. For these reasons, manna is referred to as the bread of the heavens or the food of the moon. In the Biblical scripture manna is compared with dew that is, in turn, a symbol of prayer. In the Revelation of St. John it says, "To him that overcometh will I give to eat of the hidden manna." (2:17)

In James' dream it is very clear how extraordinarily important the encounter between the unconscious and his consciousness has been for him. This would have been impossible to accomplish using any rational approach. The extent of James' wounding led me to assume that the Self had not manifested in his early childhood. In his sandplay James symbolically experienced the Self in the birth of Christ and he was given a treasure. Now he had not only the ability to learn, but he had developed a manliness that would allow him to accomplish the adaptation to the collective. One could hope that his therapy experience would lighten the storms that life might bring to James. Above all his soul was now close to God. James began to pray in his daily life, knowing that he could always seek God's help.

NOTES

18. C. G. Jung, *Symbols of Transformation*, Collected Works, Vol. 5. (New York: Pantheon Books, Inc., 1967), 180.

19. C. G. Jung, *Psychology and Religion,* Collected Works, Vol. 11. (Princeton, NJ, Princeton University Press, 1958/1977).

20. C. G.Jung, *Symbols of Transformation*, Collected Works, Vol. 5. (New York: Pantheon Books, Inc., 1967), 198.

21. C. G. Jung, *Psychology and Alchemy*, Collected Works, Vol. 12. Second Edition, (Princeton, NJ: Princeton University Press, 1953/1977), 73.

22. C. G. Jung, *Symbols of Transformation*, Collected Works, Vol. 5. (New York: Pantheon Books, Inc., 1967), 348.

CHAPTER 7

DEDE:
Speech Block
5-Year-Old Boy

Dede came to me for therapy when he was five-and-a-half years old, and treatment lasted over two years. The events that happened during this time were so varied, I have chosen to highlight just a few that were of particular importance in the boy's development.

According to his parents, Dede's blood heritage was Caucasian, Kurdish, Turkish, Byzantine, Cretan, and Swiss. This resulted in racial, cultural, and religious contrasts, among which was a mix of original ethnic culture, Islam, old and new Christianity, and regional traditions. Two of Dede's maternal ancestors had been stolen from nomad tents as small children and were brought up in wealthy Turkish families. The nomads that wandered through the steppe lived in an eternal feud with their Christian neighbors and their acts of war were based on high-level ethics of family loyalty.

I mention these details because the boy impressed me at once as being very unusual. Dede's willful, yet guileless eyes looked at me as he leaned against his mother. His vocabulary consisted of only a few words, which did not at all correspond with his age. He also exhibited other alarming symptoms. He demanded the presence of his mother at all times. He hid within her coat on the street and insisted on wearing a nightcap type of hood. He had an outspoken preference for blue and refused to wear a pullover of any other color. When asked to do anything that was against his will, Dede tensed up. Nothing could persuade him to get into a bathtub. He loved music, and he liked to draw on big pieces of brown paper. It was questionable whether he could develop in a normal way.

At the age of 21 months, Dede suffered from an acute staphylococcus infection. I learned from his treating physician that Dede's muscles were so tense, a hypodermic needle broke during an injection. This experienced doctor told me that Dede had been in great danger of losing his life for three days. He recovered relatively fast, but he was unable to walk or talk after his illness. Dede appeared to be a healthy child before the illness, but subsequently he had to learn these skills all over again. While re-learning to walk presented no difficulty, Dede's speech development lagged far behind the norm. A psychiatric report questioned whether he could even go to school. This was the primary reason the family contacted me.

Dede and I spent our first hour together in my garden with his brother, who was four years older. I observed as they played with a cable car. Dede directed the course of the game with gestures and a few words. His brother had very little to say.

The first time Dede came alone to visit me, he steered straight to the record player, indicating that he would like to hear music. Sitting on a low chair, he listened to the music intently. After a while, he motioned for me to sit beside him. We listened to Mozart. As the record finished Dede said in a very satisfied way, "Green." Then we listened to Bartok. He called this music "Yellow." I realized that these descriptions corresponded to the colored labels in the center of the records. Next he wanted "Blue." This was a Bach recording. I watched his intense listening and knew that he connected the colors with certain composers when he called them green, blue or yellow. We spent several sessions listening to these three composers. I felt that he had established a definite relationship with me, and knew that I needed to pursue additional methods in his therapy. Sitting at the piano, I played and sang a children's song. Dede moved his chair close to me and listened very attentively. I was sure that he did not miss a single sound as he sat motionless in his chair. When I wanted to turn the page and sing a new song, he emphatically prevented me from doing so. Dede loved the song about the moon, and the picture of the moon and the stars in the sky next to it. I repeated all of the verses two or three times. He did not want to hear anything else. Then he closed the book, and we went to the playroom on the lower floor. On our way we passed a gently ticking electric meter. He was startled and grasped my hand. I felt his insecurity and anxiety and assured him there was nothing to fear.

In the playroom, Dede went immediately to the sandbox. He built a hill and pierced it on all four sides with his hands, making a tunnel and a hollow space in the center. His face showed me that he did not see anything else but the cave. He discovered a candle that he put inside the cave and had me light it. Dede seemed to like this.

In the following sessions we were either at the piano or he worked in the sandbox. Dede enjoyed this. I felt that it was primarily the light in the cave that fascinated him. He molded the sand very fast and immediately brushed any remaining sand from his hands. Touching the sand seemed to be unpleasant for him.

Dede's face brightened after some further sessions. Originally he had been very serious. Now he clearly enjoyed coming. When he was picked up after his session, Dede wanted the door of my house to remain open until he had disappeared. Dede had to be sure that the house was in fact open for him. Dede began to feel close to me and would sit on my lap while I repeatedly played the "Song of the Moon" on the piano. Meanwhile, he discovered a second piece in our songbook entitled *Songs and Sounds for Children's Hearts.*[23] Woe if I ever skipped a verse! After a short while, he apparently knew them all.

One day Dede discovered paper and colored pencils. With astonishing firmness, he drew a big square. He gave me paper and pencil indicating that I too should draw my house. When I drew the door, he wanted to see it open. The old chimes beside the entrance had to be in the picture. This probably gave him the assurance that he could always come back. Dede began to feel that I understood him. Again and again he wanted to hear the songs "Good Moon, You Are Going So Quietly" and "Twinkle, Twinkle, Little Star." Each time he sat motionless and listened with great intensity.

I noticed that Dede's hearing was especially acute, as he reacted to every little noise. One day he was in my office at 11:00 am, and the church bells were ringing. He became restless, wanting me to open the window so he could hear them. I drew a church and pointed out the bells in the belfry to him. He then drew my house. In addition to the door, the drawing now had a knob that he represented with a circle. He tried to draw a bell above it. He did this in a few seconds with one stroke that radiated a tremendous vitality and sureness.

Everything Dede did was motivated by an inner necessity that left no room for alternative. His actions were dictated by his unconscious, which continued to conceal his conflicts in darkness. At the same time, something in Dede pushed towards the light. This might be the reason why the songs about the moon and the stars that lit up the sky, and the candle in the sand cave, were so tremendously important to him. Dede was interested in nothing else. At this time it would have been utterly useless to try to teach him how to tie his shoes, even though he continued to stumble over his loosely hanging shoelaces.

Two months later, just before Christmas, I showed Dede an illustration to the song, "Silent Night, Holy Night" in our song-book. It pictured a brightly lit church, some houses on Christmas night, and people holding lanterns as they walked through fields in deep snow. I sang and played the Christmas song. Dede listened attentively to the song and to the story of Christ's birth. He remembered the Christmas tree with many candles. He placed a church and a small house in the sand [Illustration 42], arranging them on a little hill. Dede no longer needed to make a cave. To complete his picture, we illuminated the church and the house with the tiny electric lights that are made for dollhouses. He thoroughly examined the church tower to see whether it contained any bells. He did not find any, but was satisfied anyway. Dede had continued to listen to the church bells ringing at noon each time he was in my house, insisting that the window be open. I wondered how he could be satisfied with our little church that had no bells, since he liked the sound so much. Because his vocabulary was still very limited, it was only later I learned he was afraid that the

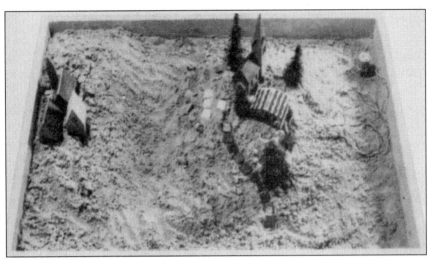

Illustration 42: Dede emerges from the darkness, as he activates his inner source of illumination.

church bells would fall down. I assured him repeatedly that there was a floor under the bell separating the bells from the rest of the belfry.

Bells are the sounds that connect heaven and earth and are a symbol of creative energies. I surmised that Dede's anxiety that the bells might drop down had to do with his fear that he could be overwhelmed by his creative energies. As he had not yet learned to cope with these energies, he wanted assurance that there was a protective floor under the bells. Knowing this presented a challenge for me to watch closely for his creative expressions and attempt to give them direction.

Dede now liked the Christmas songs with their beautiful pictures of Christmas and "Song of the Moon," as well. Again and again, he put the little house and the church in the sand. Sometimes he added a few more houses to make a little village. Sometimes the house stood alone beside the church on the hill. At times he called the house "my house" and at other times that of the Christ child. Very slowly the mother-child unity that had formed in therapy via the transference was beginning to dissolve. Dede felt completely accepted and understood and that his Self was protected. He was secure in "my house" and sometimes in that of the Christ child. I felt that his reference to the house as the dwelling place of the Christ child was evidence of the impending birth of the divine child in him. He was now ready for the manifestation of the Self.

Dede's preoccupation with the Christ child soon extended to an interest in churches. The pictures in our songbook showed the birth of Christ in connection with brightly lit churches, and Dede had already called my house a church. Enthusiastically, we looked at a book of churches and cathedrals. Amazingly well, from one visit to the next Dede remembered the names of the churches that I had shown him. He even recognized and remembered details of a certain church, because he recalled the rose pattern of its stained glass window. He continually asked me to look at the "church book," then he began to draw and paint churches himself [Illustrations 43 and 44].

Dede did not draw imaginary buildings, but real churches that he had seen either in books or during his excursions into the country. His stroke for drawing churches and cathedrals was not as sure as it had been when he first drew the square. However, what he could not say in words he seemed to be able to express in drawing and painting. I could see that an inner need was at work. He was searching for expression, as a means of communication. At times, the urgency was so overwhelming his entire being was seized by it. This may explain why no human figures appeared in his play. Dede was enthralled by something very different. Dede was fascinated at the sight of churches and by pictures of the divine birth in the stable at Bethlehem. He was equally intense about drawing and painting his churches. I wondered if it might be possible that the Christian consciousness that had lain dormant in Dede's ancestry for generations wanted to manifest in him.

Christmas passed, and another month went by. Dede continued putting the church and the little house in the sand, mostly on top of the hill. Gradually he added other houses and an additional church. There were still no people, but two white horses played in the village square. As we saw previously, the white horse often appears in connection with a religious experience. Two horses may indicate an impending manifestation of the Self.

A short time later, Dede built a pretty village on the hilltop [Illustration 45]. It is winter. Surrounded by snow-covered pine

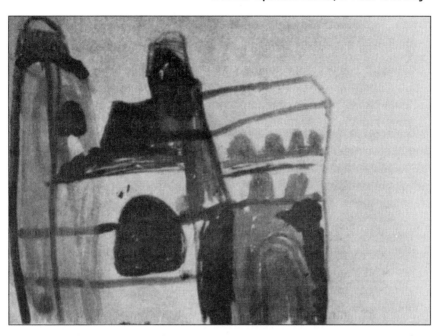

Illustration 43 (Above) and Illustration 44 (Below): Dede's religious nature awakens deep within as he passionately draws and paints churches.

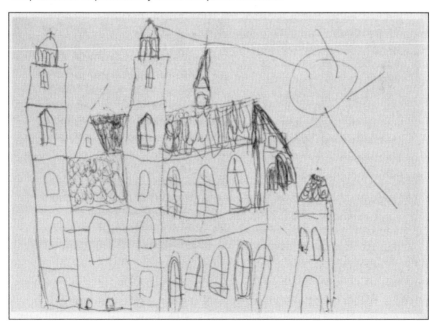

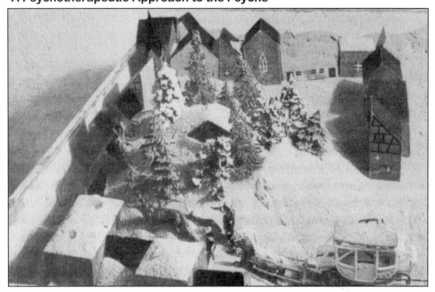

Illustration 45: Directed by his own instincts, Dede experiences a union of the opposites and the manifestation of the Self.

trees, a little wooden house and the church directly behind it stand in deep snow. A wedding carriage is drawn up the hill by both a white and a black horse. Dede remarked that it carries the king and queen. Two servants walk ahead of the coach, and leading the entire procession is a giant fox.

We had successfully restored the mother-child unity in our therapy. The alternating references to my house as the house of the Christ child indicated that the necessary separation was taking place. Dede's Self began to detach from the mother-child unity in the symbolism of Christ, the

complete, perfected human being. In this picture, the Self is represented as the union of opposites in the wedding of the king and queen and by the carriage drawn by both white and black horses. In fairy tales the fox appears when there is a need for an unconscious content to become conscious. Antoine de Saint Exupery, writer of *The Little Prince*, used the fox as the one who teaches what is invisible.[24]

Dede's intense listening to Christmas songs, the ringing of the church bells, and his drawing of churches and cathedrals, apparently arose out of the conscious awakening of a Christian tradition that had remained latent in him until now. In the form of a great fox, Dede's helpful instincts show the way to the manifestation of the Self.

Soon afterward, the ice emphatically melted and Dede began to speak normally. He was reborn. He discovered new songs in our book and loved listening to some particular ones. Dede especially liked "May Renews Everything," or "Come Dear Month of May and Make the Trees Green Again." He no longer listened with the same intensity that he had with the song about the moon, but he appeared more interested in the accompanying pictures of children at play, and of people in their Sunday outfits walking through sunny fields to church. This picture gave rise to many questions. He wanted to know everything, such as, "Why do people go to church on Sunday? What are they doing in church?" I told him they listen to stories about God that the minister tells them and that they pray and sing to organ music.

I went to the piano and attempted to improvise the walk to church and the service. I included the ringing of bells, light and heavy sounds, the entrance of the minister, the singing and the organ music. Dede was immensely fascinated and asked for repeated improvisations, until he finally tried to do the same with his own fingers. It was incredible how his clumsy little fingers labored to find the right keys, but he found them! I wondered whether he had musical talents. He now played the piano with the same intensity that he formerly used to listen to songs. He would not rest until he found the correct tune.

Dede also wanted to hear stories about God, and he listened attentively when I told him that God cares for all people. "Then he must live on the top floor," he said, "...to see all the people."

Since Dede no longer had difficulty speaking, we talked about his going to school. Normally, he would start school the following year. Throughout his entire life, Dede scarcely had any relationship with the outer world. Only under the protection of his caring parents and his older brother had he made any contact with the world at all. His parents agreed to my suggestion that he go to a private kindergarten two or three times a week, where he could meet other children his own age and get used to them. This attempt only partly succeeded.

Dede did not care at all to use his hands for crafts, as did the other children his age, and his teacher had difficulty relating to his intensity. Nevertheless, he did not dislike school and talked about the children.

Meanwhile, a different problem preoccupied him during his visits to my house. One day while leafing through our songbook, Dede discovered the picture accompanying a lullaby, "Good Evening, Good Night." I played it for him, but I do not know if he heard it. Steadfastly he looked at the baby lying in the cradle. I had to assure him that the baby lay in the cradle only during the night. He wanted to know the child's age. I explained to him that only small children sleep in cradles, and that as soon as they grow older they sleep in beds. I did not understand why he asked me these questions. He listened, and I could see he heard my answers, but he seemed to be seized by some fear. I discovered that he was worried that the child would stay in the cradle forever, in spite of my reassurance that he would not.

Instead of churches, Dede now drew cradles [Illustration 46]. I understood that he was re-living his forebodings of death, the same ones he had experienced at an early age during his illness. These great

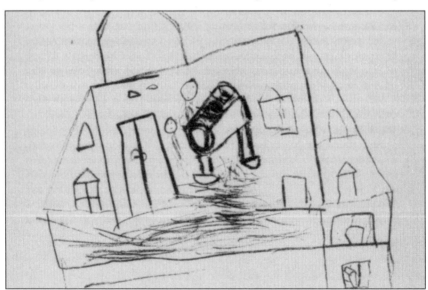

Illustration 46: Dede faces his early fears of death in his drawings of babies in cradles.

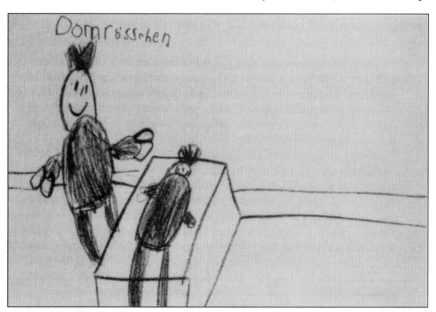

Illustration 47: Dede is fascinated by Sleeping Beauty's return to life from the confines of her glass coffin, as he accesses hope for renewed life within himself.

fears may also explain why he would not climb into the bathtub. Unconsciously he strongly feared he would be trapped. A picture illustrating the song, "Sleep, My Beloved Son," gave him a little consolation. This picture showed a mother standing beside the cradle, holding her child in her arms. For weeks Dede drew all kinds of cradles. After trying many times, he even succeeded in painting them in the right perspective. Otherwise, he made good progress.

A few months later, there was an opening in a municipal kindergarten. An intelligent teacher helped Dede make the transition to the class by allowing him to sit away from the other children to draw and paint.

During this time fairy tales appealed to Dede, especially "Sleeping Beauty." He was enthralled by the idea that the prince awakens Sleeping Beauty from a deep sleep with a kiss. In symbolic language this fairy tale gives us insight into Dede's problem, as the awakening from a deep sleep symbolizes a rebirth and the beginning of new life. Dede now drew pictures of the glass coffin with Sleeping Beauty and the Prince **[Illustration 47]**. I hoped that his old problem was slowly resolving in order that new development might begin.

The theme of renewed life became even stronger when Dede did his next sand picture. He made a broad river that many people went to bathe in. He said, "They all dive in and then come up to the surface again." Later he expressed the theme of renewal even more distinctly in a baptism scene [Illustration 48]. Dede put a small bowl into the sand and baptized a doll by holding it under water. Man and animals surround the ritual in a circle.

We know that Christ's baptism was by submersion in water. In early Christianity, baptism was a ritual that had great significance and indicated acceptance into the community. The holy water in the church today still carries this creative and transforming attribute. The experience of immersion in water was enormously important for Dede. It meant that a new life could begin that would enable him to develop the security he would need to confront the outside world.

This first step in Dede's development created a balance between the culture of his ancestors and Christianity. That the whole problem was not com-

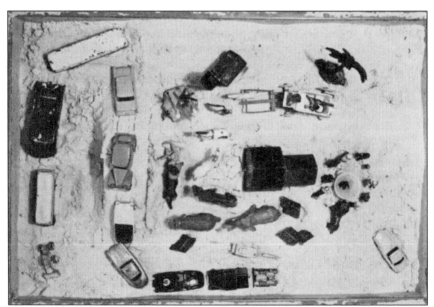

Illustration 48: Dede's wounded spirit is born anew in a baptismal ritual, as people and animals stand witness.

pletely settled soon became evident when his drawings of Christian churches began to include mosques!

Dede developed quite well. He expressed his lively imagination through his drawing and painting and played the piano a little. To my astonishment, Dede would not rest until he could play by ear some of the songs that I had played for him earlier. I am happy to say that Dede was accepted into the first grade at the normal age.

NOTES

23. *Sang und Klangfurs Kinderhez.* (Berlin: Verlag Neufeld und Henis, 1909).

24. Antoine de Saint Exupery. *The Little Prince* (New York/ London: Harcourt Brace Jovanovich, 1971).

CHAPTER 8

MARINA:
Isolation
9-Year-Old Girl

Although the small, brown-eyed girl skipped into my playroom, I saw immediately that she had mixed feelings. Her mother told her that she would come here to play. I suspected she was wondering what kind of games these would be. Nevertheless, when she saw the sandbox she rolled up her sleeves and began molding the sand. I showed her all of the figures she could use for the sandplay. With her hands on her hips, she carefully examined the shelves full of figures.

I observed Marina as she stood with her back to me. She had straight dark hair that fell almost to her shoulders. The weight of her slender, small frame was on her right leg, while the left was a little in front, balanced on the heel and pivoting from left to right. Her slightly dark complexion reminded me of the children from the Mediterranean.

"May I take whatever I like?" she asked.

"Yes, just pick the ones you like best, the ones you would like to play with most," I answered.

Marina liked a small wooden house the most, so she put it exactly in the middle of the sandbox **[Illustration 49]**. She looked at it from all sides and, apparently satisfied, turned back to the figures. She selected some trees as fencing for the grounds around the house. To the left she built a wooden fence in the shape of a half-circle. This formed a corral for a white horse that was looked after by a man crack-

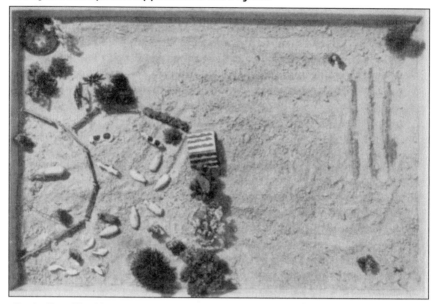

Illustration 49: Hope is sown for understanding, as Marina's longing for inner quietude assumes a central position and the white horse is ready at the hands of the trainer.

ing a whip. Domestic animals, cows, sheep, and geese grazed near the house where a girl was busy feeding the hens and geese. Marina placed all these figures precisely on the left side of the sandbox, while leaving the right side completely empty. With her left hand, she made some light furrows in the sand and set a farmer in the field whom, she said, was sprinkling seeds on the ground.

This picture represents the psychological situation that brought Marina to me for observation. Marina's adoptive mother ardently wanted a child, and she was able to adopt Marina at the age of six weeks. The small girl developed well, although she wet her bed until she was six years old. Occasionally, Marina showed strong resistance toward her adoptive parents and could be quite obstinate. When Marina was four years old she wanted a little sister, so her parents adopted a second child. Her parents lived in the U.S. and were temporarily in Europe. Since they planned to return to America in a few years, they selected a school where Marina could be taught in English, her native language. She showed

CHAPTER 8
MARINA: Isolation, 9-Year-Old Girl

a great deal of talent in drawing and handicrafts, but she had problems with arithmetic and reading. Her reading difficulties were so evident that she already required private tutoring in the second grade. The tutoring had not helped her, and her adoptive father was particularly unhappy. He had set all his hopes on an intelligent child.

The warm little wooden house has been a favorite of several children in my practice. At first it stood all alone in the center of the sandbox. I wondered if it embodied Marina's longing for a warm home, or for inner calm. It could be a desire for both. It seemed significant that the white horse grazed apart from the rest of the life on the farm, yet it was driven by a farmer with a long whip.

In mythology and folklore, the horse is able to see into the future. It is often described as clairvoyant and clairaudient. At times horses are said to have the capacity to speak. As an animal, the horse embodies an unconscious animalistic quality. As a beast of burden, it is related to what is maternal. As it is easily frightened, it is associated with the instincts and cannot be controlled by consciousness. The

symbol of the white horse also carries religious qualities. A temple is dedicated to the white horse in China. A white horse is mentioned in the Apocalypse. According to legend, Muhammad was carried by a white horse when he ascended to heaven. Additionally, in ancient religions the white horse is associated with the sun god. The horse simultaneously represents the unpredictability of nature and the inner drive toward the illumination of consciousness.

In little Marina's sand picture, the white horse is on the far left side. This probably signifies a wounded feminine, maternal aspect of the little girl, dwelling deep in her unconscious. I hoped to be able to reach this in our work. The planter on the right offers a fertile prognosis, as he casts the seed across a wide field.

To her second session, Marina brought a small bouquet of flowers she had picked along the way. When I thanked her, she said, "Isn't that nice? I love you and you love me."

"Today I want to paint," she continued. I showed her the different paints, pencils, pastels and watercolors that were available. I was astounded by the sure execution of her brush strokes. Marina developed her painting

109

into a pretty representation of a blooming tulip, which she took home to give to her mother.

During the third session, Marina occupied herself with the sandbox **[Illustration 50]**. She began by constructing a street across the sand. Then she selected some houses that she placed a little distance away from the road. The houses were Western, like those in our region. In front of the houses she made a small brook, over which she set an Oriental bridge. Next to this she placed a pagoda and, on the water, a junk. Between the Occidental houses and trees she placed some additional Oriental elements. These included small temples and a white pagoda. Marina then put large trees on the far left of her growing picture. Soon the street that stretched across the picture became populated.

With the greatest care, Marina selected all of the Oriental figures she could find, until she had enough to form a very long train of people moving from right to left. Way up in front and already disappearing into the forest is a Chinese lantern carrier. When I asked little Marina what he was doing in the woods she answered, "He has to bring light into the dark forest." I told her that she was right, for I knew that her psyche had embarked on a healing path, and I was greatly touched. Only through the dark does the path lead to light. Spontaneously and from the unconscious of a child, an eternal truth is expressed here.

In school, Marina lagged behind due to her inadequate achievement in arithmetic and handwriting. Frequently, she felt excluded from her schoolmates.

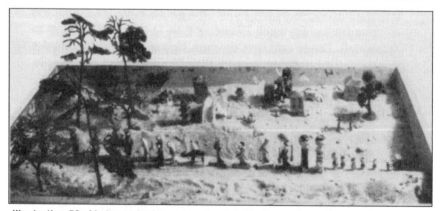

Illustration 50: Marina embarks on a journey into the far reaches of her psyche.

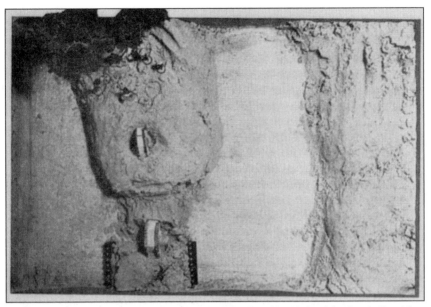

Illustration 51: The sadness of Marina's isolation is evident in her island portrait, yet the musicians who play and dance in the region of her consciousness carry hope for a brighter horizon.

Perhaps it often felt dark and lonely in her inner self. Symbolically, she had already expressed this in the first picture, in which she used the solitary, grazing white horse. It was time to find a solution to help this child move out of her inner loneliness.

The third picture was more telling **[Illustration 51]**. It represents an island that Marina called Hawaii. On the upper left-hand side of the island is a small forest. In front of this, a Hawaiian dancer and musicians stand in a semicircle and play. Below, a small round pond is crossed by a Chinese bridge. Another bridge leads to a piece of land on which stands a single, little tree. Marina's Hawaii is surrounded by water. To the far right is a completely empty field that can be seen as the mainland.

The whole thing reminded me of a very sad face. In the region of the eyes, which stand for consciousness, there are foreign musicians and the dancer. On top of this the forest looks like a tuft of hair. The small, round pond with the bridge gave me the impression of clenched lips. I saw here an expression of the entirety of this little girl's isolation. I wondered what she wanted to convey by this. I wondered if she was saying that her mouth was shut, but that she identifies herself with the dancer. Perhaps she is saying that she is a child from a far-away country, or that she feels foreign in her surroundings. Both Oriental and Occidental people live peacefully together in Hawaii. Both could be true. The secret that slumbers deep in Marina's unconscious speaks here for itself. It found expression in an external design. The bare strip of land on the right side of the picture lay nearer to consciousness. This expresses the standstill in Marina's intellectual development. Nothing grows on it. It is uninhabited. However, in the solitude she feels, perhaps because she knows she was adopted, she dances! Involuntarily, I remembered the wonderful verse of a Persian poet: "He who knows the power of dance lives in God."

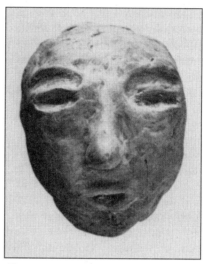

Illustration 52: Marina sculpts a dark, somber mask in clay.

I embraced little Marina for a moment to show her that I understood her language. Sharing her message together in this way communicated the full acceptance of this young girl just the way she was.

Subsequently, Marina expressed herself in many different ways. They were always creative. I was amazed by the artistic capability of this little girl. She made small shapes in clay. She colored or enameled. One day she made a little mask out of clay [Illustration 52]. At first I did not know how to interpret the mask. It was a pretty, sharply sculptured, somewhat foreign-looking little face. "It is nothing," Marina said, but I sensed that she really liked it.

In a few weeks, Marina made another sand picture [Illustration 53]. She built a hill in the center and set a church on it. At its entrance, she placed a Chinese arch. In front of the

Artistic Expectations

When I give a child clay, wood, plaster, glass, enamel, colored paper, paints and other materials, I do not expect artistic masterpieces . I use art materials and music to develop the child's emotional nature and his ability to communicate. Mainly I want to awaken the creative energy in the child. Because normal human development can only occur in relation to the wholeness of the creative center of the Self, I try to activate the inner resources that are in danger of being stunted by daily routines at school and at home. If artistic talents should be aroused by providing art materials, they will find expression of their own accord.

church, the paths divide. The path to the left leads down to a small Oriental bridge over a small brook that is shaded by blossoming trees. A little Japanese girl with a parasol stands in the middle of the small bridge. The other path heads in the opposite direction. Following a big curve that nearly forms a full circle, it leads to a village with Western houses. Situated in the right front is a small

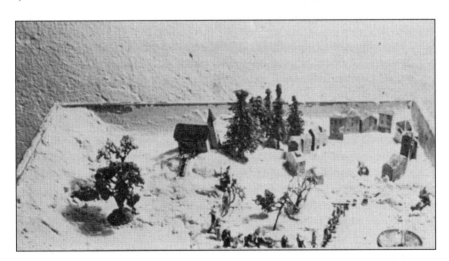

Illustration 53: Deep conflict is put to rest, freeing Marina to adjust to her adopted world.

round pond containing fish. A long train of people nears the village. They are just like the line of people that moved toward the forest in the second picture. At the entrance of the village, a little lady sits in a small rickshaw. She is the princess who is going home, Marina commented.

East and West unite in this church with the Oriental entrance. Marina knew that I understood her and could fully accept the secret that troubled her so deeply. Feeling this, she was released from the burden of her history. Her dark secret could safely return to a place of rest in the depths of her being. To be sure, a sacrifice is always demanded when a new stage of development is reached. An old situation, in this case symbolized by an Eastern element, recedes into the background to make room for a new one. In Marina's picture, the little Japanese girl takes a solitary path away from the others. Because she is represented in such an enchanting way under the blossoming tree, I felt that Marina would no longer be burdened.

It was as if East and West had met in the innermost being of the child. On the basis of this communication, the adaptation to her new surroundings could now take place with great vigor. Now Marina could begin to conform to her Western environment. She expresses this in the many people who move toward the Western-style village. The line of people moves in the opposite direction of the procession in the second picture, and now the princess is in the lead. Even the landscape with the little forest of firs has a Western character. The fish in the pond may be a suggestion of the Self in Christian terms. In order to accomplish this centering Marina has to sacrifice a part of herself. She does this directly through her little Japanese girl. For an adult, accomplishing a similar sacrifice and centering requires becoming consciously aware. The child, however, experiences this in the actual process of making the picture.

As it was summer, Marina and I often used the sunny hours for playing in the garden. The Self accompanies the entire process of development. In my opinion, the Self can be supported by the therapist through play. Marina and I frequently played a ball game on the lawn. In this game a small ball is thrown by the players to some distant point and becomes the goal. Players toss big-

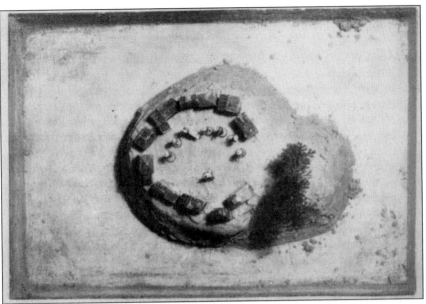

Illustration 54: New development is set in motion, as feminine energy dances in the protective womb of possibility.

ger, colored balls trying to come as close as possible to the small one. In this game, I will frequently change the starting point in order to symbolically engage the many different sides of the child, which strive toward a centering.

The play in the sand was nevertheless always attractive to Marina. After a short time, she re-created an island picture [Illustration 54]. The village from the last picture returns. Now the dancer and the musicians liven up the interior space of the village square. Even though the dancer is the only female figure in the representation, the picture indi-cates a meaningful change in the child's psyche. The dancer per-forms in a circular protected space, a kind of temenos.

Feeling sheltered is a prerequisite for all true freedom and for the freedom to develop. The difference in the quality of protection between the first island and this island is great. In the first picture, the dancer appears aban-doned and at the mercy of nature. Here she is in the protection of a man-made village that carries the archetypal character of the pro-tector in its circularly constructed form.

The incompletely closed

form of the island reminded me of the shape of the uterus and its amniotic fluid from which its fruit, the child, is released. Marina's island pictures the embryonic development that is set in motion through the mystery of dance and its dynamic. In the Great Mother, Neumann states: "Originally all ritual was a dance, in which the whole of the corporeal psyche was literally 'set in motion.'"[25]

When little Marina looked at the newly finished picture, she began to dance. She hummed a melody and seemed very happy. Evidently moved, she said, "Sometime I will dance." At the same moment she spotted our little dachshund through the window and rushed out to the garden to hug him. He liked that. Every time Marina came, she showed him her affection." He is my friend because he is so fuzzy." He was a soft, longhaired dachshund and Marina loved all that was soft and fuzzy. She also loved the rabbits our neighbor kept. Marina always wanted to feed them carrots and stroke their soft fur. I am certain she would have liked very much to take one home with her!

Marina began to behave with complete self-assurance. She was joyful and told me about her adventures. The hours she spent with me seemed short to her. She often came with a proposal about how she wanted to spend the time. I sensed that she was steadily gaining inner security.

Toward the end of the summer, Marina made a sand picture of the "Birth of Christ" [Illustration 55]. The child lay in a cave, surrounded by Mary, Joseph and the shepherds. In a lovely manner, she arranged big trees in front of them. They appear to protect the whole event. Instead of the usual three kings in the story, Marina placed four kings on galloping horses between two small, completely round hills.

I was very moved by the picture. Here Marina symbolically communicates something she could not have expressed verbally. This picture represents the archetypal birth foretold in the preceding picture. Additionally, the sheer power of it attests to her artistic gifts. In contrast to the loneliness and forlorn condition expressed in the third sand picture, we recognize that the psychic situation is completely transformed in this new birth.

The child is born in the sheltering cave, surrounded with love. Symbolically, Marina has

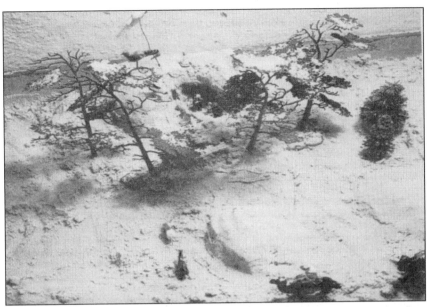

Illustration 55: Inner and outer unite in the constellation of the Self, as four kings gallop to the birth of Christ in the cave.

assimilated her despondency. Jung says of the child archetype, "...the various 'child'-fates may be regarded as illustrating the kind of psychic events that occur in the entelechy of genesis of the 'self.' The 'miraculous birth' tries to depict the way in which this genesis is experienced."[26]

The entirety of the small girl's inner experience is further characterized by the four kings that approach the cave in haste. The collective, worldly quality of these regal archetypal figures symbolizes a unification of the exterior, the world, with the inte-rior, the cave. This union happens with the constellation of the Self. This numinous, centering experience is foundational to the development of her personality and talents and for the ability to live successfully in the world. The centering experience in the sandplay arose out of Marina's unity with the therapist in a mother-child relationship.

A truly feminine aspect also belonged to Marina's personality. It seemed to me that she represented her two small breasts in the two small hills. I felt she was certainly born to be a mother.

In fact, she often spoke of how she would one day marry and have children. How right she was!

During the therapy hours, I made an intense effort to further strengthen her newly gained personality. These new-found aspects of individuality are as tender as newly sprouted grass. Happily, Marina turned with renewed ardor to artistic handicrafts. She poured a figure of a small girl out of plaster and made pretty pieces of jewelry out of enamel. She gave most of them to her mother and friends.

At this point, the problem of school reappeared. In languages and particularly in spelling, she had so far not made great progress. She had therapeutic sessions twice a week for only four months, and the time at our disposal had really been too short. Marina's father still had strong doubts regarding her intelligence. Adding to the difficulty, the second child, only five years old and also adopted, made a very clever impression.

We decided to engage a tutor who used a method suited to help Marina overcome her difficulties with reading and writing. Under her tutor's guidance, Marina wrote a short composition each day about her adventures. The words that she didn't know, or whose spelling was difficult, were written especially large and clear on pieces of paper that were arranged in alphabetical order. This way, her own little spelling book was produced. This helped Marina learn words unknown to her and to look up those she had forgotten. At first her compositions were short and consisted of simple sentences. The tutor typed out each composition and Marina made a pretty drawing to go with each one. Each sheet was carefully put into a ringed notebook, so that gradually a book of colorful stories and illustrations was made.

Marina began to show great zeal in writing and reading. Each composition gave more information about her psychic development. By the seventh hour of tutoring, she had made visible progress in reading. The following night, she dreamt that she was the best pupil in her class. She prayed to God that He might help her. The spontaneous, religious experience so impressively represented in her picture of the birth of Christ seemed to deepen in another way.

Marina formed a face out of clay that resembled Christ [Illustration 56]. If we compare

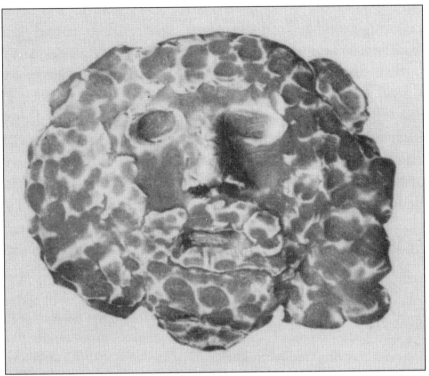

Illustration 56: Changes in Marina's Self are reflected in the placid expression of her clay sculpture.

this new face with the face she created four months before, we can clearly see the change that has taken place in her inner Self. The small figure has the features of a primitive mask, while the new face shows the calm expression of Christ.

I hoped Marina would eventually be completely free of her inner unrest, which she continued to express from time to time. One day when her little sis-

ter had had a strong reaction to a vaccination, Marina wore a sling made of her mother's silk shawl. It was frequently necessary for her to get special attention. Life was not easy for her.

Although constantly reassured by me, Marina's father did not want to believe that her intelligence was average. He insisted that she read aloud to him, which was obviously hard for her. To read to the tutor, where she and her weakness were accepted, was considerably easier. With the tutor she showed constant progress. After two months of tutoring, the great moment came when Marina could read everything that her father placed in front of her with no mistakes. Her father was touched by this long desired event. He gave a family party at once to properly celebrate the moment.

In this example, we recognize one of the motives that can lead to difficulties in the relationship between adoptive parents and children. Parents often imagine a set of pictures of the much-wanted child, and great problems arise when the child does not correspond to this image. Disillusionment on both sides is usually the result. Special empathy is required by the therapist, along with the ability to imagine himself in the environment and thought processes of both parties. In the therapy we strive for a reconciliation of opposites. This also applies to our work with the parents and children.

Marina showed real improvement. The parents decided that Marina should go to school in her native country, as they intended to return to America in the near future. In my judgment, it was too early.

Shortly before her departure, I asked Marina to make another sand picture **[Illustration 57]**. I hoped it might afford me insight into what impression the parents' sudden decision had made on Marina. Again, there is an island This time it is a mountain, crowned by a strong, compact fortress with enclosed walls. However, the tower in the courtyard is not a lookout tower, as in most fortresses. It was important to Marina that it belong to the castle's chapel. Trees and flowering bushes surround the fortress. In front of it, out in the open, stands a girl dressed in white. Below, next to the bridge that connects to the mainland, a strong man stands guard. A small ship rests at anchor.

In the early Middle Ages, fortresses and castles were built mostly on lofty heights. They afforded protection. Life and property were secure behind the enormously thick walls. When I asked who lived in this castle, Marina answered, "Mary." Since Marina had depicted the birth of Christ a few weeks earlier, it was possible to assume that the child sensed the presence of Mary, the archetypal mother. As the mother of Christ, Mary had conceived as

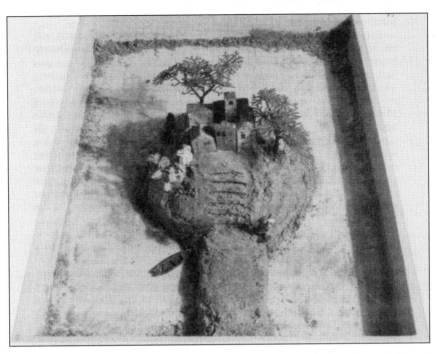

Illustration 57: Marina secures her developing inner resources in the loving protection of the archetypal mother, as she prepares to leave treatment.

innocently as had little Marina in her sand picture. As the mother of God, Mary is the essence of maternal security. This is the inner protection Marina obtained for herself. It is her own fortress that stands here. The process of Marina's psychic development reminded me of the French fairy tale, in which a white mare was helpful to a young man in mastering the difficult tasks required to win the princess. When he invited the horse to his wedding, it appeared in the shape of Mary. The fairy tale is a surprising parallel to Marina's work. Behind the walls of Marina's inner fortress, she can protect her newly acquired possessions from intruders. A guard decides who gains entrance to the fortress. This is her own inner security that she is no longer willing to surrender. Seeing this, I was hopeful that nine-year-old Marina was secure enough to face the new, still unknown, circumstances that life would hold for her.

NOTES

25. E. Neumann, *The Great Mother.* (Princeton, NJ: Princeton University Press. R. Manheim, Trans. 1955/1972).

26. C. G. Jung, The *Archetypes and the Collective Unconscious*, Collected Works, Vol. 9. (New York: Pantheon Books, Inc., 1959), 166.

CHAPTER 9

URSULA:
Depression
23-Year Old Woman

A 23-year old woman, whom I will call Ursula, consulted with me out of concern for her recurring bouts of depression. She was so depressed during the first session I knew that no verbalization of the situation would be possible. Because sandplay affords direct access to the deeper and more primitive levels of the psyche, I proposed that she make a picture in the sand. She completed the initial picture [Illustration 58] during a session of one-and-a-half hours.

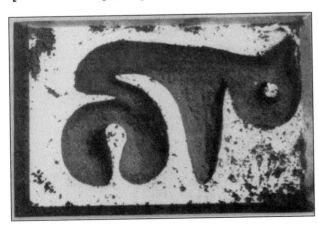

In this picture, shapes representing a uterus and a phallus lay side-by-side, bringing together symbols of the feminine and the masculine. Connected to them is a circle with a point, directed toward

Illustration 58: Masculine and feminine elements unite, as Ursula embarks on an embryonic journey to the Self.

the upper right. Overall, the form is reminiscent of an embryo. In her first sand picture, Ursula creates an expression of the unconscious sense of the opposites, as they are experienced in early childhood. With this distinctly complete representation, she initiates movement toward their union in the Self.

Ursula's contact with the sand evoked the need for her to work in clay. Three days later she sculpts the figure of a witch, who holds a sickle shaped like the waning moon. In this figure Ursula represents the archetypal negative mother, whose conquest is symbolized by the vanishing moon **[Illustration 59]**.

Ursula made a second

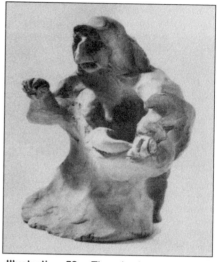

Illustration 59: The dominance of the negative mother emerges as a witch with a moon-shaped sickle. Clay sculpture.

sand picture **[Illustration 60]** two days later. In it a tree grows out of a crescent moon. Here she repre-

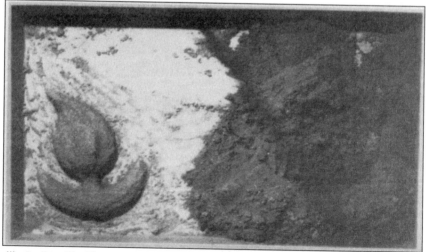

Illustration 60: The opposites unite and new growth is set in motion in the moon-shaped vessel.

124

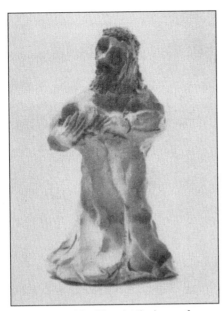

Illustration 61: The beginnings of new feminine development are embraced by the totality of the Self. Clay sculpture.

in his arms is an impressive representation of the new life [Illustration 62].

Ursula's work in the deeper levels of her psyche brought about a rebirth in the unconscious. In turn, this gave rise to the positive aspects of her own masculine component. In quick succession, Ursula produced three figures showing her positively developing masculine side. "The Prince" [Illustration 63], "The Primitive" [Illustration 64], and "A Boy" [Illustration 65]. Ursula created these figures in anticipation of the ensuing analy-

sents both the union of opposites characteristic of the Self and the powers of growth. The trunk of the tree embodies the male principle and its crown, the female principle.

Two days later, she sculpted a figure of Christ holding a crescent moon [Illustration 61]. Here the Self is represented as *imago dei*. Holding the new moon as the beginning point of new female life, Ursula's image of God establishes the basis for further development.

A subsequent sculpture of a monk holding a newborn girl

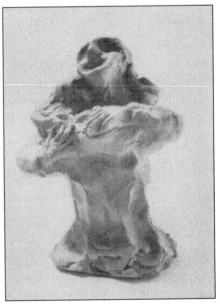

Illustration 62: A holy man tenderly holds Ursula's newly born qualities. Clay sculpture.

125

*Positive features of Ursula's developing animus
emerge in three clay sculptures
[Illustrations 63, 64 and 65].*

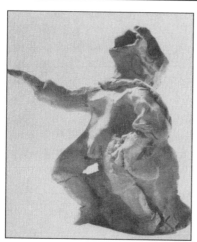

Illustration 63: *The Prince.* Clay sculpture.

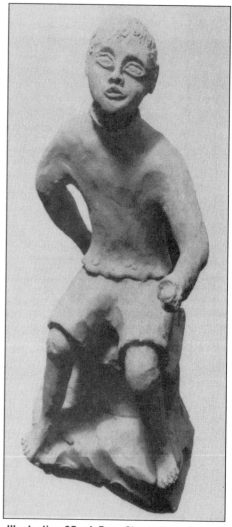

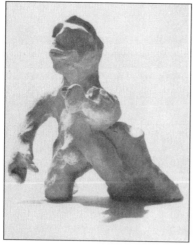

Illustration 64: *The Primitive.* Clay sculpture.

Illustration 65: A *Boy.* Clay sculpture.

sis, which would consist of bringing to consciousness and integrating her abundant dream material.

It was during the verbal analysis that we uncovered the critical moment of her developmental disturbance. As a three-year-old child Ursula made a drawing that she called a representation of man. At my request she reproduced the drawing from memory **[Illustration 66]**. It represents a urinating and defecating child, depicted by four circles. In effect, this drawing represents her early experience of the totality of man, who also has a dark side.

Inasmuch as our present culture represses the dark side of our existence, Ursula's mother called it indecent and tore it up before the little girl's eyes. In so doing, she destroyed the manifestation of the Self. Fortunately, Ursula was able to restore the Self in her analysis. This is clearly evident in the mandalas of her next two sand pictures **[Illustrations 67 and 68]**.

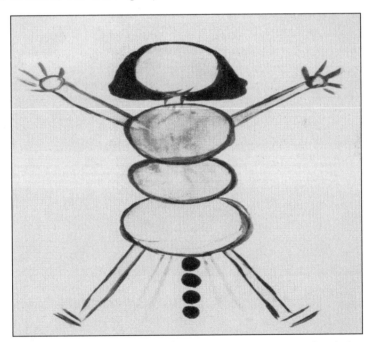

Illustration 66: As a three year-old child, Ursula experiences the wholeness of the embodied Self with its light and dark sides. Drawing on paper. Recreated from memory.

SANDPLAY:
A Psychotherapeutic Approach to the Psyche

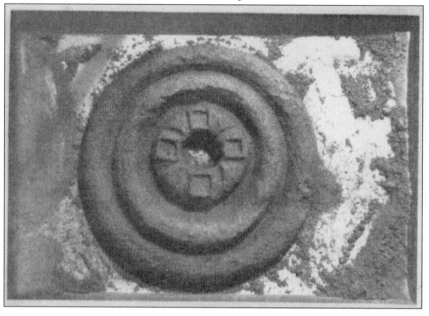

Illustration 67 (Above) and Illustration 68 (Below): Ursula restores the experience of the Self in two beautiful mandalas.

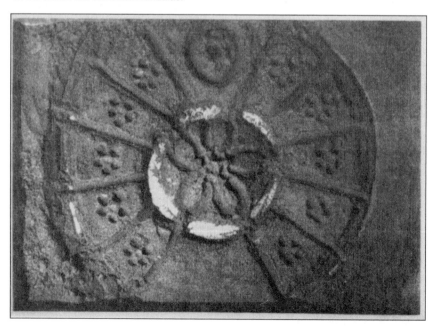

Chapter 10

Eric:

Exile

25-Year-Old Man

Eric, a young man of twenty-five years of age, asked for an appointment with me to deal with a serious case of blushing. This was a handicap in his relationships with other people and had hindered his development. Additionally, Eric was not able to decide on a professional direction. A previous verbal analysis had not resulted in the desired outcome, so he hoped to get some help from sandplay therapy.

For his first sand picture [Illustration 69], Eric looked at the

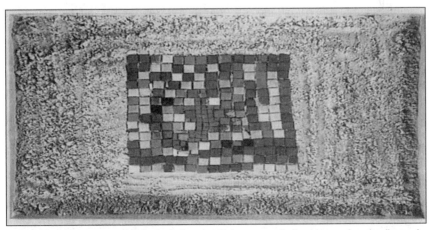

Illustration 69: An underlying religious conflict emerges in the blue, red and yellow coloration of Eric's first sandplay.

figures, but they did not appeal to him. Instead, he built a square using different shades of blue mosaics in the sandbox. The predominance of the color blue really struck me. There were only a few red mosaics near the center and two single yellow ones toward the left. It occurred to me to ask Eric what yellow meant to him. After a short reflection, he answered, "The Jews had to wear a visible yellow star on their clothing during the persecution." Eric's answer came so quickly, I deduced that he was fundamentally concerned with a religious problem. The prevailing blue color in the mosaic supports this idea. Blue is the color of the sky. It is also the color of Mary's heavenly coat. For these reasons, blue is often a symbol of the Christian religion. I wondered if there might be a Christian-Jewish problem present here.

Eric's second sand picture [Illustration 70] shows a region in Africa. This time he used some figures. Eric placed palms, a straw hut, pairs of animals, a dark female dancer and some black children. It is striking that all of the animals in this sandplay appear as couples. The number two symbolizes the contrast of polarities, as well as the tendency to connect opposites. Plato spoke of "the one and the other." As Africa is often called the *dark continent*, I concluded that his problem was still in the unconscious.

The dark-skinned dancer also indicates a side of Eric that was yet unknown to him. The prominently featured dancer in Eric's second picture is the arche-

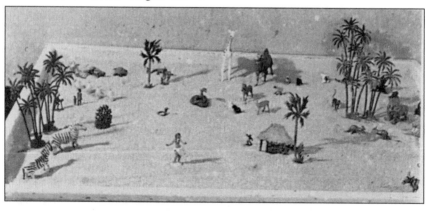

Illustration 70: Opposition and the potential for union emerge, as the still unconscious anima assumes a prominent position.

typal figure Jung called the *anima*. The anima is the feminine quality immanent in the masculine. The growing boy initially experiences the anima through the mother. The anima assumes the elementary characteristics of the maternal and is the energy that motivates the development of a young man. She unconsciously accompanies the entire process of masculine development. We can say that she animates the man's development.

Eric's third sandplay **[Illustration 71]** is an excavation site. Archaeologists are about to uncover precious floors, com-

posed of squares of golden shimmering stones. A wanderer, carrying his bundle on his shoulder, prepares to walk from the lower left corner toward the precious stones. A wanderer is a person who vainly searches for his home in the outer world, but can only find it inside himself. There is no doubt that Eric was a wanderer. He was searching for his roots and attempting to restore a lost relationship with his ancestors. Judging by his pictures, I concluded that Eric's roots were in the Near East. His pictures also told me that these roots were in the process of being uncovered.

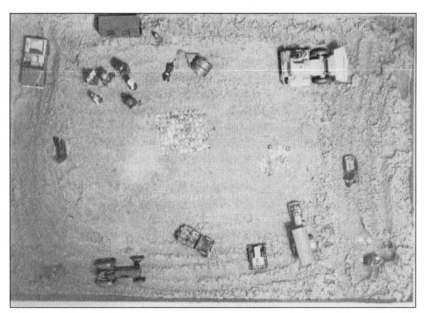

Illustration 71: Eric has a glimmer of his inner treasure, as his ancestral roots begin to surface.

SANDPLAY:
A Psychotherapeutic Approach to the Psyche

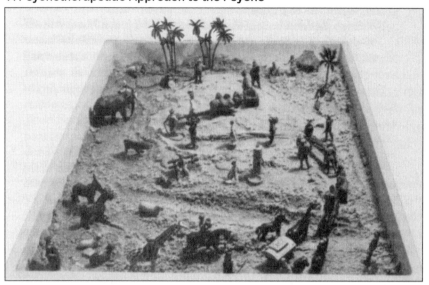

Illustration 72: Eric readies to bridge his conflict in his pilgrimage to the Self.

Eric told me that, as a young Jewish boy, he was placed in a Christian monastery to protect him from persecution. In this connection, he remembered a recent dream. He said, "In the newspaper is written, *Missing: Myself.*" Having lost his mother, Eric's longing for maternal care became overwhelming and had prevented normal development. Eric's dream shows that his ego consciousness had not formed, as a result of these circumstances. Eric's history had prohibited him from living according to his tradition in his early youth. Circumstances of history had also prevented him from ever experiencing maternal security. As mentioned previously, disturbances like these in early childhood prevent the centering constellation that leads to healthy ego development.

In his next sand picture **[Illustration 72]**, Eric builds a hill with a tree. "The Jew," Eric said, stands beside the growing tree. All kinds of people climb up the winding mountain path. There are both ill ones, carried on stretchers and healthy ones. The wanderer is on the bridge, on his way to encounter the very thing that has hindered his development. The bridge is a symbol of the connection between two poles. Eric's traveler journeys to face, "the one and the other," in the Jew at the top of the hill. Since ancient times, trees have marked the location of sacred places on elevated places. The Jew who makes a pilgrimage to Jerusalem says he "walks up the mountain." Eric's mountain symbolizes the Jewish homeland.

This young man was fulfilling the task set by his fate. He is the wanderer who joins all the other wanderers, walking up the winding mountain path. Eric shares his fate with all other people, because every human being must find the way to himself. This path leads to the experience of the divine. Everyone participates in the divine, but typically, oneness with God escapes us. Many factors contribute to people being shut off from a relationship to religion. Among them is the one-sided, rational way of thinking that developed out of the Middle Ages. Other precarious conditions such as the buffets of war, fate and exile from homelands, also deny people access to the divine nature deep within. Yet, all people are searching for the approach, the path, to this goal that is buried deep in the unconscious.

Eric shares his fate with all other people, because every human being must find the way to himself. This path leads to the experience of the divine. Everyone participates in the divine, but typically, oneness with God escapes us.

Behind the hill, children play and the dark dancer returns to dance. Whereas the dancer in **[Illustration 70]** was in the midst of conflict, Eric described these scenes as "paradisiacal." We can clearly see his development. Eric was certainly on his path to individuality, the path that each of us must travel.

After the creation of this picture, we discussed the possibility of his making a trip to Israel. It seemed to me that this trip would be help his psychic development. Even though no money was available, a "chance encounter" resulted in an invitation to visit Israel.

Before leaving, Eric made another sand picture **[Illustration**

SANDPLAY:
A Psychotherapeutic Approach to the Psyche

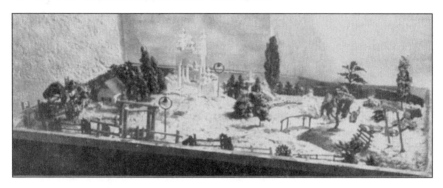

Illustration 73: "Garden of Eden." The archetypal anima is awakened, as Eric experiences centering in the Self.

73], which he called, "The Garden of Eden." A magical peace and quietude radiates from this picture. It is centered and enclosed. A gate leads to a small, artistically constructed temple. Trailing in from the periphery, rather equal amounts of blue and yellow tiles form a path to the consecrated space in the center, where a princess dances. Many cultures have traditions of walking ritual paths as a means of worship. Here Eric's search for the union of "the one and the other" brings him to a sacred procession that leads to his transformation. What appeared in the second picture as a hint of the union of the religious opposites and the transformation of the dark anima is now ready to be realized through ritual. Now the archetypal, collective anima dances in the little temple. Reaching the treasure hidden

within himself, Eric now experiences the Self. Many cultures use dance as a way of worship. For the people of these traditions the divine touches and moves them through dance. For them, dance awakens the soul. The anima activates the creative impulse in man in much the same way. When this occurs she brings true inner freedom. Of course, this level of freedom requires deep inner security. In his sand picture, the small temple and the heavenly quiet pouring forth from the garden assure Eric this security.

In my experience, the anima appears in the sand picture either at the time of, or immediately after the centering. The anima is now visible in Eric's picture. Because she manifests, we can anticipate new ego growth. As we have discussed, new ego devel-

134

opment becomes apparent following the centering. Until now, it had been impossible for Eric's ego to grow positively. The dissolution of the mother-child unity and the deprivation of maternal security had made this impossible.

While in Israel, Eric had a dream. In the dream he was looking at people who were close to a fiery volcano, and saw their skin hanging in shreds.

The shedding skin of the snake is a similar image, symbolizing transformation and renewal. In alchemy, transformation takes place in the hot fire. Fire often depicts a renewed vitality, as well. Eric's dream experience is laden with significance. When brought into consciousness, the experience of transformation and its intensified energy is often accompanied by strong emotions.

Eric truly had his meeting with the "other," in his journey to Israel. In his sandplay, Eric had

The child symbolized his newly acquired outlook on life, a transformed Weltanschauung. Eric no longer had to choose "one or the other." Now that he had experienced both, he could live with one and the other.

intuitively expressed the confrontation and integration of opposites. The actual journey allowed him to experience the process of change that had led to the manifestation of the Self. Eric now was able to look at the world in a new way.

After his return from Israel, Eric had another dream. In the dream he found a newborn baby under the branches of a great tree in a park. The child symbolized his newly acquired outlook on life, a transformed *Weltanschauung*. Eric no longer had to choose "one or the other." Now that he had experienced both, he could live with one *and* the other.

Eric described his next sand picture **[Illustration 74]** as his landing in Israel. It is a desert landscape with animals. Looking closely, I saw that the hills in the picture had the shape of a woman. She lay in the water with pulled-up knees like an embryo.

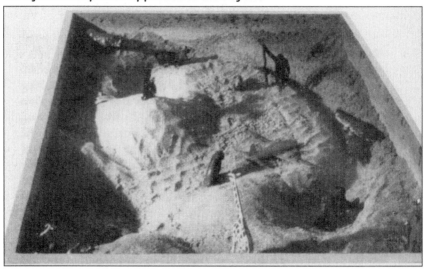

Illustration 74: Eric's personal anima is born, as he reunites with his homeland.

This was probably his personal anima, being born from the earth, the unconscious, at the moment he touched the land of his heritage. The animals of the steppe indicate the instinctual region of the unconscious. Like the ego, the anima is still on a primitive level after the manifestation of the Self. Eric's work came full circle with the gesture of her birth in this picture. The circle's point of origin had lain in the inner birth. His blushing disappeared. Soon after, he was offered a job that solved his professional dilemma and delineated a path for his future.

In his final sand picture [Illustration 75], the energies Eric will need for his new activities are released and are free to move along a wide, tree-lined path. Here, the tree symbolizes growth from the earth that unites the masculine and the feminine within itself. It corresponds to the growth and fertility of life. This path contains many colors in addition to blue and yellow, and it leads to a fruit-bearing tree. The fountain of this new life is symbolized by a well. From the well, a colorful path leads to the big, wide road. A female figure sits beside the well. She is the feminine aspect of his own being and, with her help, Eric was able to accomplish this creative work.

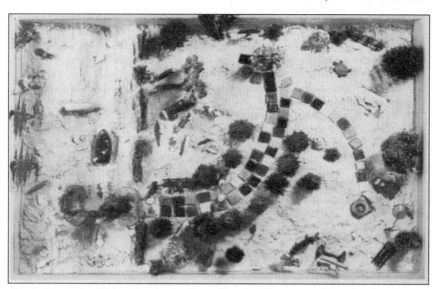

Illustration 75: Eric's anima is clearly positioned at the source of his abundant life energy. His path is now clear and fruitful.

SANDPLAY:
A Psychotherapeutic Approach to the Psyche

CONCLUSION

In the sandplay cases that we have reviewed from my practice, I have tried to illustrate how agonizing arrests in the psychic development of children and adolescents can be released, freeing the children to grow normally again. Reason alone is generally of no avail in the treatment of such developmental obstructions. This is because the many-sided psyche expresses itself in images and dreams. To access the psyche's creative center, we must try to understand this symbolic language. When we are able to understand the language of symbols, a transformation of the psyche is effected. This deep, inner transformation changes the child's entire relationship to life.

In all of the cases presented here, the possibility for achieving this higher level of development was hinted at symbolically in the patient's first picture. Sooner or later in their processes, each of these patients was able to reach the higher developmental stage. Occasionally, however, we are not successful in bringing about a new order of psychic energy in the course of therapy, and we do not achieve the expected cure.

We may encounter interruptions in treatment. It is often very difficult for the parents of troubled children to have the necessary understanding and patience to wait for a complete cure. This is particularly true because we are dealing with the irrational events of a hidden psychic process. Additionally, when signs of improvement become evident in the children after a short time, it can be especially difficult for the parents to understand the need to remain in treatment a while longer.

All in all, the course of psychic development can best be compared with *flowing water*. A commentary in the *I Ching* says:

It flows on and on, and merely fills up all of the places through which it flows; it does not shrink from any dangerous spot nor from any plunge, and nothing can make it lose its own essential nature. It remains true to itself under all conditions. Thus likewise, if one is sincere when confronted with difficulties, the heart can penetrate the meaning of the situation. And once we have gained inner mastery of a problem, it will come about naturally that the action we take will succeed.

Remember this in sandplay. And remember that when we do succeed with the work of bringing about the inner harmony that defines a personality, we speak of grace.

NOTES

The I Ching: Or Book of Changes (1950/1971). (R. Wilhelm & C.F. Baynes, Trans.). Princeton, NJ: Princeton University Press. (pp.115).

SANDPLAY:
A Psychotherapeutic Approach to the Psyche

TABLE OF ILLUSTRATIONS

SANDPLAY:

A Psychotherapeutic Approach to the Psyche

TABLE OF ILLUSTRATIONS

SANDPLAY:
A Psychotherapeutic Approach to the Psyche

SANDPLAY:
A Psychotherapeutic Approach to the Psyche

TABLE OF WORKS CITED

CH	NO	CITATION	PAGE
1	1	C. G. Jung, *Symbols of Transformation*, Vol. 5, Collected Works. (New York: Pantheon Books, Inc., 1967).	1
	2	E. Neumann, *The Child.* (New York: G. P. Putnam's Sons, 1973).	1
	3	F. MacKenzie, *Chinese Art.* (New York: Marboro Books, 1961).	4
	4	R. Kellogg, *Analyzing Children's Art.* (National Press Books, Palo Alto, CA, 1970).	5
	5	J. H. Pestalozzi, *Wie Gertrud ihre Kinder lehrt*, in Jung's Collected Works, Vol. 9. (Zurich: Racher, 1945).	8
	6	C. G. Jung, *Psychology and Religion, General Remarks on Symbolism*, Vol. 11, Collected Works. (New York: Pantheon Books, Inc., 1963),191.	8
	7	J. J. Bachofen, *Mutlerrecht and Urreligion* (Leipzig: Kroner, 1926).	8
	8	R. Bowyer, *Lowenfeld World Technique: Studies in personality.* (New York: Pergamon Press, Inc., 1970).	9
	9	E. Neumann, *The Child.* (New York: G. P. Putnam's Sons, 1973).	10
	10	M. Lowenfeld, *The Non-verbal Thinking of Children and its Place in Psychology.* (London: The Institute of Child Psychology, 1964).	16
2	11	C. G. Jung, *Psychology and Religion: East and West*, Collected Works, Vol. 11. (New York: Pantheon Books, Inc., 1963), 276.	31
	12	E. Neumann, *The Child.* (New York: G. P. Putnam's Sons, 1973).	32

SANDPLAY:
A Psychotherapeutic Approach to the Psyche

CH	NO	CITATION	PAGE
3	13	C.G. Jung, *Psychology and Religion: East and West*, Collected Works, Vol. 11, (New York: Pantheon Books, Inc., 1973), 193.	42
	14	Lao-tse, *Tao-te-king, Das Buch von Sinn und Leben*, translated and annotated by Richard Wilhelm, Eugen Diederichs, (Dusseldorf/Koln, 1957).	43
	15	E. Herrigel, *Zen in the Art of Archery*, (New York: Pantheon Books, Inc., 1953), 12.	46
4	16	*I Ching, Book of Changes*, R. Wilhelm & C.F. Baynes, Trans., (Princeton, NJ: Princeton University Press, 1971), 115, Hex. 29.	58
	17	W. F. Otto, *Menschengestalt und Tanz* (Munich: Hermann Rinn, 1956).	60
5	-	No Works Cited	-
6	18	C. G. Jung, *Symbols of Transformation*, Collected Works, Vol. 5. (New York: Pantheon Books, Inc., 1967), 180.	77
	19	C. G. Jung, *Psychology and Religion,* Collected Works, Vol. 11. (Princeton, NJ, Princeton University Press, 1958/1977).	80
	20	C. G.Jung, *Symbols of Transformation*, Collected Works, Vol. 5. (New York: Pantheon Books, Inc., 1967), 198.	85
	21	C. G. Jung, *Psychology and Alchemy*, Collected Works, Vol. 12. Second Edition, (Princeton, NJ: Princeton University Press, 1953/1977), 73.	86
	22	C. G. Jung, *Symbols of Transformation*, Collected Works, Vol. 5. (New York: Pantheon Books, Inc., 1967), 348.	89
7	23	*Sang und Klangfurs Kinderhez.* (Berlin: Verlag Neufeld und Henis, 1909).	95
	24	Antoine de Saint Exupery. *The Little Prince* (New York/ London: Harcourt Brace Jovanovich, 1971).	100
8	25	E. Neumann, *The Great Mother.* (Princeton, NJ: Princeton University Press. R. Manheim, Trans. 1955/1972).	116
	26	C. G. Jung, The *Archetypes and the Collective Unconscious*, Collected Works, Vol. 9. (New York: Pantheon Books, Inc., 1959). 166.	117
9 - 10	-	No Works Cited	-

150

SECTION	CITATION	PAGE
FOREWORD	Lowenfeld, M. (1979/1993). *Understanding Children's Sandplay: Lowenfeld's World Technique.* Cambridge: Margaret Lowenfeld Trust.	vii, xii
	Mitchell, R.R. & Friedman, H. (1994). *Sandplay: Past, Present and Future.* London: Routledge.	xi
	Montecchi, F. (1993). *Giocando con la sabbia: La psicoterapia con bambini e adolescenti et la sandplay therapy.* Franco Angelli.	xiv
	Weinrib, Estelle L.(1983/2003) *Images of the self: The sandplay therapy process.* Cloverdale, CA: Temenos Press.	xiv
	Archives of Sandplay Therapy. Edited and published by: The Japan Association of Sandplay Therapy.	xi
	Journal of Sandplay Therapy. Sandplay Therapists of America.	xi
	Magazine for Sandplay-therapy. Publishing house sandplay-therapy, Landauerstr. Vol. 16, D-14197 Berlin, Germany. (pp. 166)	xi
CONCLU-SION	*The I Ching: Or Book of Changes* (1950/1971). (R. Wilhelm & C.F. Baynes, Trans.). Princeton, NJ: Princeton University Press. (pp.115).	140

SANDPLAY:
A Psychotherapeutic Approach to the Psyche

INDEX

M

SANDPLAY:
A Psychotherapeutic Approach to the Psyche

SANDPLAY:
A Psychotherapeutic Approach to the Psyche

SANDPLAY:
A Psychotherapeutic Approach to the Psyche